D0732227

The
Caregiver's
sourcebook

The
Caregiver's
sourcebook

Frena Gray-Davidson

Contemporary Books

Chicago   New York   San Francisco   Lisbon   London   Madrid   Mexico City
Milan   New Delhi   San Juan   Seoul   Singapore   Sydney   Toronto

Library of Congress Cataloging-in-Publication Data

Davidson, Frena Gray.
   The caregiver's sourcebook/by Frena Gray-Davidson.
     p. cm.
   Includes bibliographical references and index.
   ISBN 0-7373-0136-8 (alk. paper)
    1. Home nursing. 2. Caregivers. 3. Care of the sick. I. Title.

RT61.D38 2001
362.1'4—dc21   2001028903

Contemporary Books

A Division of The **McGraw·Hill** Companies

1 2 3 4 5 6 7 8 9 0 AGM/AGM 0 9 8 7 6 5 4 3 2 1

ISBN 0-7373-0136-8

This book was set in ITC Galliard and Gill Sans
Interior design by Brenn Lea Pearson
Printed and bound by Quebecor Martinsburg

Cover design: Cheryl Carrington
Cover photo: The Stock Market

McGraw-Hill books are available at special quantity discounts to use as premiums and sales promotions, or for use in corporate training programs. For more information, please write to the Director of Special Sales, Professional Publishing, McGraw-Hill, Two Penn Plaza, New York, NY 10121-2298. Or contact your local bookstore.

This book is printed on acid-free paper.

Dedication

This book is dedicated to the memory of David J. Wenner,
anthropologist, 1920–1998, a gentle man who loved
good food and bad dogs.

Also to Joe and Olga Floren and Clar and Yvonnne Zink,
for being wonderful examples of how good friends
and caring neighbors can make a huge difference
in difficult times. Thank you.

Contents

Acknowledgments   ix

Chapter 1

Becoming a Caregiver   1
   Accepting the Challenge • Daily Problem Solving •
   Developing a Plan • Establishing Comfort Levels •
   Remember Emotional Comfort • Making the Home Safe
   • Patient Checklist • Caring for the Caregiver

Chapter 2

Common Conditions That   29
Require Long-Term Care
   Parkinson's Disease • AIDS and HIV • Cancer
   • Alzheimer's Disease • Stroke • Heart Disease

Chapter 3

Professional Resources   53
   The Doctor • HMOs and Hospitals • Pharmacists •
   Home Health Services • Hospice • Mental Health
   Services • Hiring a Professional Caregiver • Choosing a
   Nursing Home

Contents

Chapter 4

Paying for Health Care   69
Entitlement Programs • Medicare • Medicaid •
Navigating the System • Tips for Choosing an HMO
or a Managed Health Care Plan • Private Insurance
• Other Sources of Money

Chapter 5

Legal Responsibilities   87
Legal Documents • The Patient's Legal Rights
• Elder Abuse • A Caregiver's Responsibilities

Chapter 6

Death Comes as the End   101
The Predeath Vigil • Death Away from Home
• The Dying Process • One Last Checklist • Grieving

Appendices
    A. Finding In-Home Services   111
    B. Caregiver Education   121
    C. Internet Resources   127
    D. State Agencies on Aging   131
    E. State Hospice Organizations   141
    F. Long-Term Care Ombudsman and   145
       State Survey Agencies
    G. Alternative Resources to Enhance Home Life   149

Glossary of Terms   153

Bibliography   155

Index   159

Acknowledgments

It would not have been possible to complete this book without the help of research consultant Helen Saul, Ph.D., whose patience is legendary, command of the Internet masterful, and dedication to duty admirable.

I would also like to acknowledge the help of Geocities, which carries my Web site, and of Karen Largent at Suite 101. She has used her spare time to create a wonderful source for caregivers.

Finally, I want to acknowledge the Holy Trinity Benedictine Monastery, in Saint David's, Arizona, which gave me a peaceful place to write much of this book.

Thank you all.

CHAPTER 1

Becoming a Caregiver

Two-thirds of all Americans are involved in looking after someone else—a family member, an older friend, a neighbor down the street. Some people even give up their jobs or work shorter hours to look after an ailing family member. We hear a lot about how selfish people are, how people no longer look after one another. But this is not true. We are a caregiving society. And whether you are a family member, a volunteer, or a professional caregiver, my purpose here is to offer you both practical information and emotional support.

There is nothing as decent as one human being caring for another. This is the essence of how we should live. Together we are like a tribe, protecting one another, accepting responsibility for one another. We reach across the barriers of race and language and religion when we help to fulfill the needs of others. It can almost be said to be sacred work—this reaching out—because the sick, disabled, or aged person demands the best of us on a daily basis.

It is a challenge to touch and be touched on such a deep level. Your own deep issues about love and need will constantly be stirred. As you begin to care for another person, you also begin to discover things about yourself. And this is a blessing. But wanting to care for another person is not enough. Generally speaking, if you do not care for yourself, or about yourself, you cannot care properly for someone else. There is probably no worse fate for a sick person than to be looked after by an angry, overtired caregiver who is preoccupied with her own personal problems. I hope you will find support in this book for your own journey as a caregiver, and I urge you to stay alert to your own personal growth. Caregiving can transform your life—often in very unexpected ways. If you have the potential for this work, you may even find that it offers spiritual rewards.

And our society needs caregivers. Today, more people than ever before are living into old age. People survive illnesses and accidents in greater numbers than at any time in history. We are also facing new plagues that often require home care. AIDS and the newly emerging autoimmune diseases—fibromyalgia, lupus, chemical sensitivity, and Gulf War syndrome—all are on the rise. We are also in the middle of an epidemic of cancer. One woman in nine has breast cancer and one man in four has prostate cancer. At some point, most of these people will need home care.

There has never been a more urgent need for people to learn the art of caregiving. And yet there are few resources to teach us this art. We are trying to learn in a society that has temporarily forgotten these necessary skills.

There are several reasons why this is so. After the Second World War, health care became institutionalized. People would go to the hospital if they were seriously ill. Old or sick people who needed long-term care would go into the appropriate institutions. Death, and birth, no longer took place at home.

In the past few years, changes of lifestyle and economics have meant that most people, even mothers of small children, work outside the home. The increasing divorce rate, coupled with falling levels of child support, have left many women, the traditional caregivers, in a difficult position to do the job. Generally, neighbor women no longer help at birthing. Relatives no longer nurse their elders. It is not even easy for some women to be available for their own children.

The average American has no experience in caring for others at either a birth or a death, let alone helping at a sickbed. This would seem astounding to our ancestors, and even to people from other societies today. We seem to prefer that our life passages take place secretly, away from inquisitive eyes.

Luckily, things are beginning to change, and we are starting to gain a new perspective. More and more men attend the birth of their children. People who are gravely ill more often remain at home, embracing the inevitable cycle of life and death. Yet most people are out of practice in the arts of attending at a birth, or caring for someone in sickness or in his final days.

As a strange side effect of the human potential movement, caregiving has even become tainted in many people's eyes. In our drive for personal growth and self-development, we as a society, and as individuals, may have spent considerable time identifying unhealthy patterns of caregiving in our families. Sometimes we are too co-dependent, caring for others in self-destructive ways. At other times, we avoid the whole issue of caregiving completely by leaving it out of our lives. Our children are in kindergarten, our parents in care homes.

I believe that we now have the psychological tools to reshape family life and help wounded individuals to heal. We must not forget in our housecleaning that caregiving itself is noble and necessary, and that it needs to be taught well. We need people with these skills now, and we will need them especially in the future.

Today, high-tech care is the fashion in medicine—miracle surgery, powerful drugs, drastic interventions for serious diseases—but following treatment, the patient is usually sent home as quickly as possible. Generally the people at home are not equipped to look after her, and they need help immediately. Nowadays most long-term medical care is limited to brief consultations with doctors, who are usually not well versed in the practice of hands-on caregiving. So I believe that caregiving education must become commonplace, and that caregiving itself—already necessary—must become fashionable.

As a caregiver, you will learn mostly through trial and error, and through experience. But by the time you really know enough, unfortunately, you may no longer need the knowledge. The purpose of this book, therefore, is to try to help you to learn as quickly as possible, so that you can put your knowledge to immediate good use. I also wish to put caregivers in touch with other people and resources that can help and support them.

The depth of concern people can show for one another, once they know what to do, is astonishing. I hope that this book will inspire you to the wonderful work that caregiving can be.

Accepting the Challenge

Remember the instructions we receive on a commercial airline? In case of emergency, says the flight attendant, your oxygen mask will drop down from the ceiling. If you are traveling with a dependent person, put your own mask on first. Then help the other person.

A lot of the information in this book will be about putting your own oxygen mask on first. The biggest barrier to good caregiving is the caregiver's reluctance to do this. Self-destructive sacrifice is not noble, and you will not find it sanctified in this book. The emphasis here will be on your responsibility to look after yourself before you can look after anyone else.

Even if you find yourself forced into caregiving when a family member suddenly needs your help, you can still go about it in a healthy way. But to do this, it is crucial not to think of caregiving as martyrdom. It must not be a wound to suffer or a cross to bear. People who ask "Why me?" are opening the door to disturbing questions that cannot be answered.

Things happen. They just do. No one does it to us. God does not decide to strike people down with accidents. God does not hand out illnesses like pieces of poisoned cake. Reasons beyond our knowing affect the changes in our lives. Why does a person get cancer? Because of heredity, environment, life events, food, stress, and many other factors. Some of these factors we can control; some we cannot. Why do accidents happen? Usually because someone has been careless, or because a particular coming together of events brings a person into the wrong place at the wrong time. Danger and disease are omnipresent in our haphazard universe, and we humans are the victims of this chaos.

The real point is not why or how things happen. I believe that the person who asks "Why me?" is usually saying something quite different. He is really saying, "I don't want to deal with this!" This is an understandable reaction, but it doesn't help us if it leads us to avoid doing what is necessary. Instead, we must get the knowledge we need to cope. A better question might be "How will I learn to manage what I am asked to do?" A better question still is "How am I going to grow?" Once you can ask yourself this question, you are already on the road to healthy caregiving.

If you find yourself confronted with taking care of someone you did not intend to help, you have two choices: Either try to take care of him as best as you can, or do not take care of him at all. Even if you think there is no one else to do the task, in fact someone else can usually be found.

In many states there is an official called the Public Guardian who is charged with looking after the welfare of those who have no one to care for them. The state will often make sure that these people have a place to live, nursing care, clothes, and even pocket money.

So sometimes you are not indispensable as a caregiver. There is nothing worse for a dependent person than to be looked after by an impatient, resentful, or blaming family member.

But while most of us do not relish the task of becoming caregivers, neither do we wish to abandon the person who needs care. So we tend to buck up and do the job, learning as we go. There are some hidden rewards in becoming a caregiver, but only if we cast away all reluctance and embrace the task wholeheartedly.

Caregiving leads to the heart of everything that matters. It is a form of meditation in action. Caregiving can heal your own wounds and losses by encouraging in you a flow of unconditional love, which envelops both you and the person you look after. Furthermore, caregiving is a challenge if you are looking after someone whom you do not particularly like. It forces you to come to grips with issues of tolerance, patience, and forgiveness.

You begin to realize what really matters and what does not, sometimes working in the shadow of death. If you are present for the coming of a death, you will experience mysteries that no words can convey. This experience must be lived through long days and nights of watching and assisting someone who is dying.

I believe you may come to understand that death need never be feared. By helping someone through this great passage, you may even transform your own life. Once you have been present at someone's end, you may learn not to squander your own precious time.

I believe that the highest spirit of human evolution reaches to us across the centuries and stirs our better nature. As you sit with a sick old man or woman, you may truly experience that person as "all our Grandparents"—as the Native Americans say.

It is easy to forget that we are all a part of something greater than ourselves—the expanding human river of birth, suffering, death, and transformation. Every day we live reflects this universal truth—we are part of the essence of all the life that has passed before.

Caregiving is not a lowly job, as some people may think. It is not a limitation on the life you want to live. It is actually the opposite. Walking with someone on the road of suffering, following along to the gate of death itself—this is heroic. I believe that we have not honored enough this hero who is a caregiver.

In the rest of this chapter, I discuss some of the things you will need to know to meet the challenge of caregiving.

Daily Problem Solving

A competent caregiver should have a plan for dealing with problems as they arise. Caregivers can easily become overwhelmed, so it is essential to establish a daily routine to minimize disruptions. But before I get into routines, it is useful to remember the wise Chinese saying, "When you can't change a situation, then you have to change your mind."

Not all problems have ready solutions. Some problems must simply be lived with, and this is a challenge. Ask yourself, "Whose problem is this?" Sometimes the problem is partly yours. Sometimes you can solve the problem by being adaptable and accepting.

A woman whose husband was increasingly disabled by Parkinson's disease was upset when he couldn't climb the stairs to his bedroom. A visiting nurse suggested that a sitting room downstairs be converted into a bedroom for him. This idea upset the woman, who refused to consider having a downstairs bedroom. So the problem became a daily source of distress for all concerned. The man had to be dragged up the stairs by his wife—with both of them at great risk of falling. This nightly ordeal made the wife more upset than ever.

If someone had asked "Whose problem is this?," the issue could have been clarified. The initial problem was the man's disability, but his wife's refusal to adapt made everything worse. It would have been much easier for both of them to cope with the disability if the husband could have had his bedroom downstairs.

Were there other hidden issues? Did the wife want her husband gone? Was she in denial about the real state of his health? Did the downstairs bedroom remind her of their early poverty? It's a mystery why she was so stubborn, but the ultimate problem was hers.

"Whose problem is this?" A caregiver must face problems directly by asking that question. It is common for caregivers to make life harder for themselves, so honesty is essential. Once you decide whose problem it is, you can find a solution.

The first problem for everyone concerned is learning to accept the disease. People who are seriously ill go through the emotional stages identified by Elizabeth Kübler-Ross in her classic book *On Death and Dying*. (This book is primarily about patients with a terminal illness, but much of it is applicable to other patients as well.) These stages are anger, fear, denial, acceptance, resolution, and peace. Like the patient, the family caregiver goes through these stages. Many problem-solving difficulties are connected with the caregiver's inability to deal emotionally with a loved one's disease.

If you understand these emotional stages, you can better analyze your own mixed feelings. Those feelings are common to everyone in your position. You are in a process of adaptation. Go easy on yourself, so that you don't get stuck emotionally.

Be careful not to put yourself in the position of fighting someone else's disease. This is a sure way to destroy your own peace of mind. Learn all you can about the disease, and learn how it typically affects the patient. Know what to expect. That way, your sympathy will be at the highest level. Then allow your acceptance to be realistic. This doesn't mean that you should give up all hope, but fantasy is not beneficial to anyone.

Dorothy's husband has Alzheimer's. She tells him not to answer the phone. He does answer it. She gets angry with him. Once she really understands that he cannot remember her order, she is able to let go of the issue and instead gets an answering machine and turns off the phone's ringer. By understanding Alzheimer's and not taking it personally, she manages.

Don's wife has had a major stroke. Since the stroke, she cries very easily. Sometimes Don fails to remember that his wife's crying is an aftereffect of the stroke. Her sadness makes him sad, but he needs to stop getting exasperated with her. She needs to feel more emotional support from him. Don must learn to cope better.

We can never fully control our feelings or our responses. We may be feeling helpless, angry, or desperate—but we need to accept these emotions so that we can live with them. This is exactly what therapists are for. Do not hesitate to seek therapy for yourself if you have trouble dealing with your own emotions. To help your patient, you must understand your own feelings first.

You also need to be well informed about a disease so that you can make the right decisions for your patient. This should be obvious. For example, Millie has Alzheimer's. One day she wakes up in what seems to be an unusually bad mood. At breakfast she starts throwing dishes around—something she has never done before. Her husband, Phil, knows enough about Alzheimer's to realize that no Alzheimer's patient suddenly gets worse overnight or experiences major behavioral changes from one day to the next. Therefore, he takes Millie to her doctor. The doctor runs tests and discovers that Millie's real problem is a bladder infection.

Sue's Dad has terminal cancer and lives in a nursing home. One day he seems extremely confused and starts picking fights with the staff. They call Sue, and she calls her father's doctor. The doctor tells Sue that her father has obviously developed Alzheimer's and needs to be in an Alzheimer's care unit. Sue is a nurse, so she doubts this diagnosis. She takes her father to the hospital instead. There it is discovered that his potassium levels are wildly imbalanced. The imbalance is caused by his cancer, not by Alzheimer's. The hospital treats him, and he becomes calm and rational again.

In both these cases, if the caregivers had not been well informed, they would not have made the appropriate decisions. If you want to solve problems, learn as much as you can about the patient's disease.

Developing a Plan

You need to develop a plan for caring for the patient. To do this, you must keep records. First, make sure that you have all the details you need concerning the patient's medical care—even in an emergency situation. This includes all official documentation, notes about drugs that the patient is taking, and the telephone numbers of all the patient's doctors and other concerned parties. Put all the information into a special file and keep it near the telephone. If you have a helper, make sure that that person knows where this file is and how to use it.

The file must also contain all documentation concerning the patient's final wishes for treatment, including a copy of medical directives and a living will. If you hold power of attorney for health care decisions, that must be in the file too. You will take this file to the hospital in case of an emergency.

If your patient has stated that there will be no resuscitation, and all documentation to this effect has been signed, one copy of each document must be filed with the attending doctor. Remember that in an emergency you cannot call 911 and then prevent them from resuscitating the patient. Emergency medical teams must follow their procedures, which include reviving anyone in need, even patients who appear to be dead.

Developing a plan also means discussing the probable "end scenario" with the patient's doctor. You need to be ready for death care at home. Ask the doctor what you will need to do and make sure you have all the medications necessary to keep the dying patient comfortable. If you have a helper, be sure that that person is fully informed as well. The helper should be both willing and able to cope with a possible end scenario also.

Be sure that you know how and where to get help to deal with new medical problems. If the patient's mobility becomes affected, if pain intensifies, or if the patient needs a different diet, know that there are solutions to all these problems. Here the doctor's nurse may be your best resource. Ask for help. Don't hesitate to say "I don't know how to feed my mother now that she can't swallow well." Very often the answer is obvious only to a professional. For example, a person who has had a stroke may have trouble swallowing thin liquids. Adding a thickening agent, such as gelatin or baby gruel, will help the person to swallow without choking. Nurses know this, but a family dealing with the situation for the first time may have no idea what is going on or what to do about it.

In any case of medical difficulty, write down what is happening and describe it exactly to the patient's doctor. She may ask you to bring the patient in, or she may refer you to a dietician, a nurse, or a physical or speech therapist.

If the physical equipment you have is not working for the patient, ask the doctor where to get what you need. Medicare supplies a wide range of equipment. Sometimes you must take the initiative. One ninety-seven-year-old woman had a major stroke and became totally disabled. Her doctor made no suggestions for her rehabilitation, thinking that at her age she could not recover. When her family members learned from their own research that rehabilitation might help, they reapproached the doctor. He prescribed it. The old woman recovered nicely and lived for another year. During that year, she was able to live much more comfortably than she would have otherwise, thanks to the physical rehabilitation.

Establishing Comfort Levels

An excellent way to monitor your progress as a caregiver is to begin each day by monitoring levels of physical comfort in the person you care for. Consider pain, stiffness, aching, ease of movement, ability to change position, clothing, bedding, bowel conditions, skin, and so forth. No matter what the problem is, there is always a solution. No one needs to stay in pain these days. Although there are still some cultish beliefs about pain, most doctors want the terminally ill to be free of it.

Make a checklist. It might include the following steps:

- Encourage the patient to take pain medication. These days this does not mean being drugged or spaced out. Ask the patient's doctor to prescribe an appropriate dose. If you are dealing with a hospice, it will be much easier because hospice personnel are skilled at managing doctors and drugs. Doctors all too often undermedicate terminally ill patients, leaving them in pain. National surveys confirm this. Hospice nurses are more skilled in pain medications and therefore can intervene in getting them adjusted.
- Encourage the patient to take a good laxative early in the day. Doing so can prevent the misery of constipation, although drinking a lot of water usually does the trick even better.
- Massage is helpful for a sore body. Hire a professional.
- Many clothes worn in everyday life are simply not comfortable for a sick person. Dress the patient in soft cottons and loose clothes, warm socks, and possibly no underwear. Most people who are really ill do not resist these changes.
- Keep the bed comfortable. Use sheepskin to soften it and egg crate mattresses to ease soreness. For protection against

bowel or bladder leakage, use plastic under the bottom sheet, or dress the patient in incontinence wear. Many of these things are covered by Medicare if the patient's doctor will prescribe them. Some insurance covers them also.

- Keep the room as light and bright as the patient can stand.
- Play nice music.
- Place fresh flowers in the room.
- Use essential oils such as lavender, orange, geranium, and lemon to scent the air. Add two or three drops of lavender to wash water to calm and refresh the patient. If skin is chafed or sore, you can rub it on directly. For more about essential oils, see appendix G.

Remember Emotional Comfort

What is the level of emotional comfort in this caregiving situation? If the person you care for is profoundly angry, frightened, hopeless, or lonely, this will make life harder for both of you.

- Find a way to talk about problems, if possible.
- If the patient will not talk about her emotions directly, perhaps you can casually mention worries and indirectly inspire her to open up to you. To do this, you must be subtle.
- If there is unfinished family business, try to find ways to close it. If you don't know how, perhaps a therapist can help you by suggesting possible approaches.

Most sensitive people are concerned with the "great questions." People without any type of spiritual practice may be more troubled than others, since they may actually feel more alone. Some issues that cause emotional pain may have a spiritual basis. Examples include fear of death, rage at being picked out by an illness, regrets over the way one has lived, and doubts about one's place in the universe. It will take courage for you to approach emotional issues with sensitivity. Be aware that the patient may be unwilling to discuss these things. It is always best to remain calm and centered. Remember that your peaceful, helpful presence is enormously valuable in itself.

Your own emotional comfort is important, too. You may feel overwhelmed by some of the problems that you face in caring for the patient. But almost any problem of this kind can be solved if one knows where to look for the answer. The appendices in this book list many sources of information. Write down the names and numbers of useful people whenever you meet them or talk to them on the phone. These names will become part of your permanent resource list. Don't feel embarrassed to call anyone with your concerns. That's what people in the helping professions are there for.

If you are caring for someone with a specific condition, it's important to learn how his disease is likely to affect his behavior, as I have already explained. Not only will this help you not to blame the patient when life becomes difficult for you both, but—most importantly—it will ease your fear. For more on this topic, see chapter 2.

Finally, never assume the worst. We never really know what will happen. You might read about Alzheimer's disease and picture your husband lying helpless in bed. This is a very depressing picture. Yet in reality, only about one patient in thirty-five ends up like this. So again—never assume the worst, even though it is normal to fear it.

Hope is the most effective medicine. A cure may well be found for any disease. Back in the early 1920s, people with diabetes routinely expected to die young. Then insulin was discovered, and literally overnight this fatal disease was transformed into a merely chronic condition. We are now seeing progress even with AIDS, as more people live longer with HIV.

Hope is vital to life. Don't give up hope.

Making the Home Safe

The following checklist suggests ways in which you can make the home safer for the patient.

Floors
- Replace or remove loose rugs.
- Do not use throw rugs.
- Replace loose linoleum or tiles.
- Cover uneven thresholds.
- Use nonskid rugs in bathrooms and kitchens.
- Move all electrical cords away from traffic areas.

Stairs
- Remove all clutter from the stairs.
- Install adequate lighting for stairs.
- Replace a worn or frayed stair covering.
- Install sturdy handrails on one or both sides of the stairs.
- If the patient cannot climb the stairs, install a ramp or a chair lift.

Kitchen
- Keep most-used or favorite dishes within easy reach.
- Use plastic or unbreakable dinnerware and glasses.
- Turn the handles of pots and pans away from the edge of the stove.
- Keep hot pads and oven mitts within easy reach.
- Wipe up spills as soon as they occur.
- Have a fire extinguisher within easy reach, and know how to use it.
- Depending on the patient's mental condition, attach a stove guard and childproof knob protectors, so the stove cannot be accidentally turned on.

Bathroom
- Use nonskid rugs on the floor and skid-resistant mats in the bathtub.
- Install grab bars by the toilet, bathtub, and shower.
- Install adequate lighting, and keep a night-light burning constantly.
- Install faucet handles that can be turned on and off easily.

Outside
- Remove all tripping hazards, such as hoses, garden equipment, and vines.
- Remove debris, such as snow and leaves, from sidewalks.
- Repair damaged steps or sidewalks.

Security Systems
- Install smoke alarms.
- Install carbon monoxide alarms.
- Purchase personal safety and medical alarms and put them in place.

Patient Checklist

Here are some ways to keep your affairs organized and ease the daily demands of caregiving:

- Make sure that the patient's legal and financial affairs are in order, and that you know where to find the relevant documents.
- Make sure that the patient keeps his medical and dental appointments annually, or more often if needed.
- Make sure that the home environment is clean, safe, and pleasant.
- Make sure that the patient's needs for good exercise, sleep, and social activities are being met as well as possible.

- Attend to the patient's personal hygiene and grooming needs daily.
- Make use of respite services at least once a month.
- Review the patient's level of care once a month to ensure that she will be able to remain in the home.

Caring for the Caregiver

"He's getting better," says Judy after her husband's stroke. "I look after him—but who looks after me? That's what I want to know."

Many caregivers probably feel like asking the same question. The fact is that if you are a caregiver, the one who must look after you is you. Your peace of mind rests in your own hands. It is a tragedy when caregivers neglect themselves, and this tragedy gets played out every day. As one caregiver said at a workshop, "I just don't have time to take care of myself." Beware of this sentiment, because there is nothing noble about it. Most often it means that you are angry and frustrated. A caregiver who punishes herself with an overload of work usually has a poor self-image.

Caregiving is demanding because it touches you at the deepest level of personal relationships. It involves not only intimacy with the patient, but also your inner security in dealing with others. People who have unresolved issues about love, or who suffer from feelings of worthlessness, or who carry deep wounds left over from childhood are sometimes drawn to become caregivers. Ironically, your ancient pain may be exactly what enables you to help others. You may understand where to find deep personal healing because you have experienced it yourself. But this, of course, implies that your own issues have been resolved. Caregivers whose issues have been stifled or ignored may become unconscious abusers. They may abuse the patient. Or they may abuse themselves.

You must acknowledge your emotional issues and deal with them. You don't want to become a menace to yourself and others. If you are overtired, you can make terrible mistakes, mistakes that may be life threatening. You can incur injuries—back injuries or torn muscles, for example—that never fully heal. Under stress, you can make awful remarks that will haunt you forever.

There are many reasons why you may forget about yourself. Ill people often need you suddenly, and that can be unsettling and overwhelming. Because there is so much to learn, to do, to remember, you stop paying attention to yourself. You must be constantly alert to your own stress levels and emotional needs. You must provide yourself with physical and psychological nourishment.

Some caregivers don't think their own needs have any value, so they treat themselves with neglect. These caregivers may be unwilling to admit that they are not coping well, so they won't ask others for help. They think "I should keep my troubles in the family." But sometimes this is a way of holding on to control.

Caregivers can get depressed. They can become too exhausted to do a good job. Their stresses make them nervous and overwrought. They cannot nurture the patient or themselves.

Cheryl lived next door to her mother, who had mild dementia and needed daily help from her daughter. Cheryl was angry at the situation and was verbally abusive every time her mother made a simple mistake, such as putting on the coffeemaker without filling it with water.

When a friend challenged Cheryl about her attitude, Cheryl cried, "You don't understand how terrible it is to see someone you love fall prey to an illness like this!" But screaming abuse at her mother was not a sign of love. It was a sign of rage and fear. Cheryl's mother had been a perfectionist and had raised a daughter who was nervous, easily overwrought, and unable to nurture. Of course, the mother herself had never been nurtured, so she was unable to teach Cheryl this skill.

Cheryl desperately needed therapy, but she was unwilling to seek help. Her sick mother suffered for this—the result of a sad parent–child relationship that went back fifty years. Clearly, there was a complex psychological history in this relationship.

Overwhelmed caregivers are incompetent caregivers. They make poor decisions and create a loveless atmosphere that makes the patient's last journey in life lonelier and more painful than it needs to be.

At the Holy Trinity Monastery in St. Davids, Arizona (where I stayed while I was working on this book), there was a sign on the dining room notice board that read: "Blessed are the flexible, for they shall not be bent out of shape." This could well be the prayer for every caregiver. Learning to be flexible is one important key to dealing with the feeling of being overwhelmed.

It Helps When You Know What to Do

I once lived with a ninety-seven-year-old woman who did not need a lot of care—just someone around the house. It was an easy life for awhile, since she lived in a pleasant part of the Berkeley hills in California. Suddenly she had a major stroke, and I had to become a full-time caregiver of a very different kind than I was used to. I was scared and ignorant. What should I do? Would I kill her accidentally out of ignorance? How would I get her to the bathroom? How would she eat?

For a few days, I was totally overwhelmed. I could neither eat nor sleep. But eventually some visiting nurses taught me what I needed to know. We even called in extra help. Things got better. I began to sleep again. Gradually things fell into a smooth pattern. I realized that the old woman was in her last days, but the experience of looking after her became enriching. It was constant work until she died, but I was seldom overwhelmed again.

You will feel much less overwhelmed once you know what to do. Getting the information from the nurses helped me the most. Have a nurse come in and teach you the skills that you need. Pay the cost out of your own pocket if it isn't covered by Medicare, Medicaid, or the patient's insurance. It will be worth the money.

I learned in one afternoon the technique of turning a completely helpless patient in bed. I learned how to feed her, and then how to deal with her bowel and bladder eliminations. I learned what her possible end might be, what complications to expect, and how to deal practically with her death when it came. It certainly took a while to absorb all this and feel competent—and I had my own emotional issues to struggle with—but the nurses' openness got me on the right path.

Once you know what to do, obtain any special equipment that you need to help you do it. Ask the patient's doctor or the home health nurses what is available. There is special equipment now for everything, including lifting someone out of bed or into a bath. There are many types of wheelchairs. There are breathing and exercising machines. You can even find special enema kits. All this technology will make your work easier.

Sleep

You must get enough sleep. This is another place where flexibility comes in, because sometimes caregivers have to catch sleep whenever they can. If you can't get a good night's sleep, grab naps in the daytime, or sleep when the patient sleeps, even if it's in the morning or afternoon. If you cannot catch up, you must call in someone else to give you a break. There must be no exceptions to this rule. Caregivers who don't sleep can quickly become anxious, despairing, and suffer serious breakdowns in health.

How can you induce sleep? Essential oil of lavender often helps—two drops on your pillow, three drops in your bathtub, diffused with a diffuser in your bedroom. Other herbs that may help you to sleep are valerian and passiflora (passion-flower). Both are available in tincture form from your local herbalist or natural health store. (Follow directions on the packet.) Many people swear by Calms Forté, a mixture of homeopathic herbs.

Nutrition

You cannot get by on junk food snacks and soft drinks. Caregiving is a high-stress job, so you need a good diet. Try to cook properly for yourself. If you simply do not have the time, buy food that is nourishing and requires no cooking. Examples include fresh fruits, dried fruits, nuts, yogurts, cheese, soy milk, good breads, good crackers, and gourmet soups. Get a dip or spread to eat with freshly chopped vegetables, or hard-boil some eggs and keep them in the refrigerator.

Don't drink too many sodas or too much caffeine. If you are under a lot of stress, try eating six small meals a day. Take vitamins. Make a point of sitting down when you eat, even if you're only eating a snack. Give yourself a break so you can digest your food in peace. If the stress causes you to lose your appetite, blend yourself a protein drink from fresh fruit, yogurt, eggs, and honey. Sip it slowly. These fruit and vegetable smoothies are very nutritious.

Cook large meals and freeze them in small portions so that you will be supplied for awhile. If someone asks if you need help, ask her to cook something for you. Be sure to tell her which healthy food you like most. It can be anything from a casserole to a cake. Most friends and neighbors are thrilled to help out in this way.

Exercise

It's crucial to get enough exercise. Your body needs it, and it helps your emotions too, by lowering stress. One traditional

Chinese remedy for depression is to take a good, brisk walk. This helps when you feel agitated, upset, or angry, as well. If you cannot leave the house and there is no one to relieve you, walk briskly in place.

You can do other kinds of exercise at home. Try aerobics, yoga, or tai chi. Nowadays you can get great videos to help you along. Do gentle stretches whenever you feel yourself getting stiff. Be careful about doing sit-ups or touching your toes, unless you are already in good condition. Reach out your arms, gently swing them at shoulder height, gently rotate your ankles, and stretch your legs. Take it easy. All this works.

Safety Precautions

When you're lifting the patient, always take care to bend your knees. And always move in close. Find a professional to show you the proper way to lift someone. Use belts or supports to help you, if necessary.

When turning someone in bed, use a sheet beneath his body to move him. Don't strain your own muscles—especially your back muscles. It is better to lower the patient temporarily to the floor than to risk slipping. Call your local emergency service when you need to. Don't be embarrassed. They're glad to help. They would rather help you to move the patient safely than take both of you to the hospital.

Proper Breathing

Oxygen is what people under stress need most. Make it a point to sit at least once an hour and take ten slow, deep breaths. Breathe from deep in your lower belly up through your lungs. Don't be surprised if you immediately become more aware of how you feel. The relaxation will make your body more sensitive, and the breathing will clarify your consciousness. These breathing exercises will help you to cope better, even to sleep better.

When you feel especially stressed, add four drops of oil of lavender to your bath and deeply breathe in the aroma. It may calm you and help to create a sense of peace.

Know the Warning Signs of Fatigue

As a caregiver, you cannot afford to get sick yourself. Fatigue lowers your resistance to illness. The following are signs that you are seriously fatigued:

- You can't get to sleep. You awaken at 3:00 A.M. and can't get back to sleep. You fall asleep finally, but when you wake up, you are tired.
- You have aches and pains throughout your body.
- You experience a resurgence of previous ailments, such as allergies, skin problems, digestive problems, or arthritis.
- You are exhausted, or conversely, you are unable to keep still. You are hyperactively busy.
- You are forgetful and cannot concentrate.
- You lose emotional control at inappropriate times.
- You feel fearful, anxious, and worried all the time, often without knowing why.
- You cannot reach out to or communicate with others.
- Your muscles are tense, and headaches won't go away.

If you find yourself experiencing any of these symptoms, watch out for yourself. Don't convince yourself that you'll feel this bad only until a problem is over. That is the biggest lie we tell ourselves. Start feeling better now by taking better care of yourself.

Emotional Health

Caregiving is sometimes an ordeal. It's normal to react emotionally when you're going through an ordeal. You may become angry at yourself, at other people, at the person you're caring for. You may wake up in the middle of the night, staring at the ceiling, terrified. You may cry too much. You may not cry at all, yet wish you could. You may become resentful and needy. Anger, fear, and grief are normal responses to a difficult situation, so don't condemn yourself if you feel like this.

Once when I was very angry at someone, I wrote his name on a piece of paper. Then I jumped up and down on the paper. It may sound childish, but it made me feel much better. Another way of dealing with your emotional reactions is to ask yourself, "How did this person really hurt me?" Writing it out helps reduce the stress of holding everything inside. Meditating, which is designed to lower stress, can also help to improve your emotional health. There are lots of tapes and videos that can teach you how. The object is to bring your mind under your own control, to become calm and clearheaded.

Try to retain your sense of humor. That's one of the best ways to get through any crisis. Spend time with someone you can tell the terrible things to. Seen from a different perspective, those terrible things may start to seem funny. Everyone who works on the edge appreciates graveyard humor. Emergency crews constantly tell grisly jokes to survive the terrible things they see and do. You might try renting comedy videos, especially if you've begun to think you may never laugh again.

Handling Grief

It's natural to grieve if you are losing someone you love. Give way to grief; to do so will ease your feelings and take toxins out of your body. Eventually the grief will run its course. It is only those who suppress grief who can't move through this natural process. This is not to say that the loss you feel will ever be completely resolved. Any loss has a permanent echo, and we should honor that. But you can adjust so that your life will still have meaning and joy. Your task now is to make everything manageable, and to survive.

The main way to do this is to share your pain with someone. Find a friend you can really talk to—perhaps someone who is dealing with a similar situation. But don't forget to give that friend equal time for his own problems. Or you may wish to see a therapist. Most therapists can recommend support groups, and these can be very comforting, too.

If you have a spiritual practice, follow it wholeheartedly. If you are a member of a spiritual community, share with them and take all the help they can give. I recommend that you avoid people who tell you that everything is God's will. God doesn't kill people for the sake of our spiritual development. Things just happen. Sometimes they happen to people we love, and we hope God is there to help us through the ordeal. We would like to believe that He is and be soothed by that belief.

Nowadays many sources of support are available via the Internet. The immediacy of E-mail makes it easy to reach out from your home and share your feelings with other people across the globe. The more caregivers communicate, the better we all are for it. It is always surprising who turns up in a crisis. Old friends may sometimes let you down, but strangers may reach out when you least expect it.

When someone close to you is dying, should you actually think about caring for yourself? Yes! Since you will probably not have the time to do many things you like, make a list of activities that you would enjoy if you could. Taking a long, hot soak in the tub; getting a massage; going out to a movie; building something in your yard; having a drink; reading a novel; playing cards or bingo or chess; getting your hair styled; taking a walk in the park; going fishing; going shopping just for yourself; buying yourself flowers; getting an afternoon's sleep with no interruptions—these are just a few suggestions to get you started.

Now pick three things from the list that you could do every day. Plan how you are going to do them, and stick to this plan.

Understand that it's okay to enjoy yourself even if someone is dying. In fact, it's essential—but it won't happen if you don't make it happen. Find somebody to look after the patient while you take a break. Ask your friends, ask your neighbors, ask the members of your church. Ask a relative. Hire someone if you have to. But make time for yourself.

People who say "If I can do anything, just let me know" usually mean it. Tell them, "Why yes, now that you mention it, I could really use a couple of hours off. Would you sit with my mother on Wednesday?" If they back away, don't push it. But if they agree, make sure they know all they need to know about the patient's condition.

Make the patient comfortable before you leave and give him his medication so that nothing will spoil the afternoon. If you make things easy for your helper, she may help you out again. Leave all the phone numbers she might need—the doctor's, the home health worker's, and your own. You might suggest an activity to pass the time. Perhaps she could read a book or watch a movie with the patient. You may not wish to go out; perhaps you will simply use your free time to stay home and catch up on lost sleep. Perhaps you'll take that long, hot, soaking bath you've been promising yourself.

Make time for yourself. Use it as you like. Do this on a regular basis. Everyone will benefit. You can use the following checklist as a guide.

The Caregiver's Checklist
- I am getting out or exercising at least once a week.
- I am getting seven to nine restful hours of sleep a night.
- I talk with or visit three friends or relatives a week.
- I see my doctor and my dentist once a year.

- I check a new resource on caregiving each week.
- I am eating balanced meals every day.

Learning to be a caregiver can be a challenge. But if you follow the suggestions in this chapter, meeting that challenge will be the most rewarding thing that you have ever done.

CHAPTER 2

Common Conditions That Require Long-Term Care

It would not be possible in one short book to discuss all the medical conditions that require intensive home care. In this chapter, I will discuss only the six most common ones. These are Parkinson's disease, AIDs and HIV, cancer, Alzheimer's disease, heart disease, and stroke.

I am neither a physician nor a medical expert, so this chapter is intended to give you only very general information concerning these conditions. For an in-depth analysis, you should see a medical professional or seek out clinical information in bona fide medical texts.

Caregiving is empathy. The more we understand the specifics of a person's suffering, the better able we will be to find the best way to help ease it.

Parkinson's Disease

Parkinson's disease is a slowly progressive, chronic condition that affects a small area of cells in the midbrain known as the substantia nigra. Gradual degeneration of these cells reduces dopamine, a chemical in the brain.

It is estimated that up to 1.5 million Americans are affected by Parkinson's disease. Although 15 percent of these patients are diagnosed before age fifty, Parkinson's generally targets older adults. While there is as yet no cure for this condition, current treatments allow many patients to live almost normally throughout their lives.

The following are classic signs of Parkinson's disease:

- A resting tremor that occurs on one side of the body
- General slowness of movement (bradykinesia)
- Stiffness of limbs, rigidity
- Walking or balancing problems (postural dysfunction)
- Small, cramped handwriting (micrographia)
- Inability to swing the arm easily on the affected side
- A decrease in normal facial expression (hypomimia)
- A lowering of volume in the voice (dysarthria)
- Strong feelings of depression and anxiety that have no obvious cause
- Immobility when initiating a step (freezing)
- A slight dragging of the foot on the affected side
- An increase in scalp dandruff
- Oily skin
- Inability to blink the eyes
- Difficulty in swallowing

Few patients exhibit all these signs, and some may exhibit signs that are not listed here.

Parkinson's disease should not be confused with Parkinsonism. This is a separate condition with Parkinsonlike features. It is usually caused by drugs that interfere with the brain's metabolism of dopamine. Chief culprits appear to be phenelzine (Nardil), tranylcypromine (Parnate), and some kinds of antihistamines. Check with the patient's physician or a pharmacist for specific details.

Medications most often prescribed for behaviors of Parkinsonism, which can include dementia, are haloperidol and other drugs used to treat hallucinations and confusion in the elderly; some antihypertensive drugs that contain reserpine; and a commonly prescribed antinausea drug called metoclopramide (Reglan).

Parkinson's disease often begins with an intermittent tremor of the hand on one side of the body. The patient may be distressed by the tremor because other people can see it, but this sign rarely leads to serious disability. Resting tremors may be accompanied by slowness and stiffness on the affected side. As these signs progress, patients may notice impairment on the other side of the body, but this impairment is usually less severe.

Motor deficits may become more pronounced. Finger and hand movements requiring skilled coordination—such as brushing teeth, shaving, and buttoning clothes—become difficult. Some patients develop a slight foot drag on the affected side, and walking requires a great effort. Steps become shorter, and freezing of movement may occur. The patient's voice may gradually become soft and difficult for others to hear. As the volume decreases, the voice may also take on a rasping quality.

It is important to stress that the nature and severity of these signs varies greatly from one patient to another. It is rare when a patient experiences all of them. Parkinson's disease is not a fatal illness, although the physical incapacitation may frighten the patient and make him believe that he is about to die. This is especially common when the patient experiences balance problems. Anxiety is compounded by the difficulty of navigating doorways and narrow passages; the tiny, jerky steps the patient must take; and the constant struggle for balance.

Preventing falls and injuries is a top priority for both the patient and the caregiver. If the effects of Parkinson's interfere with the patient's ability to manage her daily activities, a physician may recommend physical, occupational, or speech therapy to address the specific problems.

Counseling for patients and caregivers can be helpful as well. Stressful adjustment reactions, anxieties, or depression can arise in the family living with Parkinson's disease. The spouse, children, and friends of the patient need special attention and guidance. There are networks of support groups throughout the world for patients and their families. To locate the group nearest you, contact the National Parkinson's Foundation.

Medical Management

A knowledgeable physician can offer patients much in the way of medical management and supportive therapies, especially if she is compassionate and sensitive to the patient's many needs. Parkinson's patients must be candid when describing their symptoms to the physician in order to get the full benefit of the doctor–patient relationship.

Many signs of Parkinson's can be controlled with currently available medications. Levodopa (also called L-dopa), the active anti-Parkinson's drug in Sinemet and its generic brands, is the medication that is most often used. Levodopa is a short-acting drug that enters the brain and is converted into dopamine, the neurotransmitter that is deficient in Parkinson's patients. Levodopa is combined with another drug called carbidopa, which enhances its action in the brain and minimizes side effects, such as nausea. (Approximately 12 percent of patients experience mild nausea with Sinemet, but this nausea usually subsides after a few weeks.)

Amantadine (Symmetrel) is an antiviral drug that also provides an anti-Parkinson's effect; it is most frequently used to widen the therapeutic window for levodopa.

Benadryl, Artane, and Cogentin are brand names for anti-cholinergic agents that may be prescribed to treat tremors. Although they are effective, these drugs can have side effects, such as dry mouth, blurred vision, urinary retention, and constipation, which limits their use in older adults.

Bromocriptine (Parlodel) and pergolide (Permax) enter the brain directly at the dopamine receptor sites and are often prescribed in conjunction with Sinemet to prolong the duration of action of each dose of levodopa. They may also reduce levodopa-induced involuntary movements, called dyskinesia.

Dyskinesia can be tricky to diagnose in the Parkinson's patient. It may be symptomatic not of Parkinson's disease itself, but of Parkinsonism, which is a drug-induced condition. One typical sign of drug-induced dyskinesia is an involuntary movement of the tongue, sometimes combined with drooling. Parkinson's patients should be monitored for dyskinesia on a regular basis.

Medications used singly or in combination can significantly enhance motor performance and treat other symptoms of Parkinson's disease. Unfortunately, there is currently no medication that will prevent or cure it.

Nutritional Guidelines

Parkinson's disease slows the functioning of the digestive system. Swallowing is prolonged, the stomach takes longer to empty, and food passes through the intestines more slowly. Food should be eaten in small amounts and eaten frequently. Try six small meals rather than three large meals a day.

If the doctor has prescribed Sinemet, most Parkinson's patients will derive more benefit from it if they take it on an empty stomach. They should take it at least fifteen minutes before a meal (thirty minutes is better) with four or five ounces of nondairy fluid. This will wash the pill from the stomach through the pylorus valve and into the small intestine, where absorption begins.

If Sinemet causes nausea, a small cracker or a bite of fruit can be taken with doses between meals. Pretzels are excellent, because they are portable and require no refrigeration. Ginger can also be used to offset nausea. Have the patient drink ginger ale, or give him a piece of ginger root to chew.

Only a small percentage of Parkinson's patients need to alter the amount or timing of protein intake to avoid interfering with Sinemet absorption. These are patients who experience significant on–off motor fluctuations and who typically take Sinemet six or more times per day.

It is hard for many Parkinson's patients to maintain their weight. Taking frequent, small meals may help. Liquid supplements can also be useful. Sometimes patients are so diligent in limiting fat intake and worrying needlessly about protein restrictions that they deprive themselves of needed calories.

Although most dietitians consider supplements unnecessary if a person eats a variety of foods, some health care providers view a daily vitamin and mineral supplement as a nutritional insurance policy. The patient should not be given megadose vitamins, however. Any supplements should be taken with food. It has been theorized that free radicals promote Parkinson's. Antioxidants, including vitamin C, may help to combat this process.

The natural sense of thirst may diminish with age, putting elderly people at risk of dehydration. Anti-Parkinson's drugs dry out the body and increase this risk. It is important for the patient to drink lots of water and to drink it on a regular schedule, maybe once an hour.

Checklist for the Parkinson's Patient

Here is a list of other things for the Parkinson's patient to do and for the caregiver to be diligent about:

- The patient should consciously lift his feet to counteract the slight foot drag common to Parkinson's disease. In this way the patient avoids shuffling and reduces the risk of falls.

- The patient should avoid prolonged standing with his feet too close together. This too increases the risk of falls.
- For better balance executing turns, the patient should avoid the instinctive pivot maneuver. She should practice reversing direction by using a forward-facing wide u-turn.
- If balance is a problem, the patient can learn to use a cane with a large rubber tip. This takes practice, but once mastered, the classic walking stick is portable, affordable, and invaluable.
- If the patient's feet feel frozen or glued to the floor when she starts to walk, she can break the pattern by stepping over an imaginary obstacle or rocking from side to side. It is not helpful for the caregiver to pull the patient forward or to tell her to hurry up; this will often prolong the freezing episode.
- The patient should swing both arms freely when walking. This may require a deliberate effort, since the automatic nature of many movements is diminished in Parkinson's. Gently swinging the arms helps to maintain balance and lessens fatigue.
- Trying to do two things at once may cause problems. Formerly automatic reflexes may work less efficiently if competing sensory stimuli take the patient's attention away from a motor function. For instance, it may be difficult for him to walk and talk at the same time. For this reason, the caretaker should minimize distractions.
- If the patient has difficulty getting out of a chair, he should place his feet directly under his knees and stand up firmly, using the large thigh muscles, rather than pushing himself up with his hands and arms. Practicing this maneuver strengthens the quadriceps muscles and helps to maintain independent movement.

- The patient should not wear rubber- or crepe-soled shoes, since they grip the floor and may cause tripping.
- Patients who experience a tendency to fall backward or to feel lightheaded should move slowly when changing positions. They should sit on the side of the bed for fifteen seconds before standing, and stand in place with support for another fifteen seconds before they start to walk.

AIDS and HIV

AIDS, a deficiency of celluar immunity induced by infection with the human immunodeficiency virus (HIV-1), is transmitted in very limited ways. The cause of AIDS and HIV is still unknown, although both are generally believed to be caused by one of a group of viruses carried in the body fluids. It has been demonstrated repeatedly that AIDS and HIV are passed from one person to another only through the transfer of body fluids. Thus these diseases are almost always transmitted in one of three ways: through sexual contact, through the sharing of intravenous needles, and through transfusions of contaminated blood.

It is also possible to contract these diseases if one has open wounds and those wounds come in contact with the patient's body fluids. In rare cases, some health care professionals have contracted AIDS by accidentally sticking themselves with an infected needle. In general, however, caregivers and others in close contact with these patients need not worry about being infected, as long as they observe simple precautions. Hugging is totally safe. Just don't handle or come into any contact with the patient's body fluids—blood, feces, urine—except under sterile conditions and with proper protection. If the patient is incontinent or has open wounds, or if there is a chance that you will come into contact with his body fluids in any other way, you must consult with the attending physician about the appropriate precautions to take.

Since HIV and AIDS cause a breakdown of the body's immune system, the patient is generally unable to fight off secondary infections. Weight loss often follows when these opportunistic infections become established in the weakened body. As the body grows weaker, the AIDS becomes more secure, and so a vicious cycle is set in motion.

Infections associated with HIV include viral infections, such as Epstein-Barr; bacterial infections, such as tuberculosis; community-acquired infections, such as *Streptococcus, Staphylococcus,* and *Haemophilus;* and fungal and parasitic infections. Adrenal insufficiency, or inadequate production of adrenal hormones, can be caused by certain anti-HIV/AIDS drugs, by the HIV infection itself, and by some opportunistic infections. Adrenal insufficiency can result first in fatigue; then in weight loss; then in hypotension and dizziness; and ultimately in death.

Decreased testosterone production is common in HIV-infected men. Like many of the adrenal hormones, testosterone helps to regulate mood, sexual function, nutrient metabolism, and energy levels. Over 40 percent of men who are HIV-positive have low levels of testosterone. Among the various causes are some of the drugs used in treatment.

Inadequate hormone production may also contribute to anemia. This can occur in HIV-positive people with normal kidneys, but it can be more severe in people whose kidneys have been damaged by HIV itself.

Medical Management

Today, various medications appear to be keeping many HIV patients from developing full-blown AIDS. However, many drugs used to treat HIV infection or its complications also have toxic side effects that can lead to anemia. This likelihood increases as immune function becomes progressively impaired. Among the drugs commonly associated with anemia are AZT (Zidovudine, Retrovir), TMP/SMX

(Bactrim, Septra), ganciclovir, dapsone, pyrimethamine, interferon, and cancer chemotherapy.

Some AIDS patients take anti-inflammatory drugs to combat the infections associated with weight loss. Commonly used anti-inflammatory agents include aspirin, ibuprofen, and naproxen. Anti-cytokine agents include pentoxyfylline and thalidomide.

It is important to remember that although many of these drugs have potential side effects, they may be essential to the patient's therapy. The caretaker should be aware that side effects may occur and should discuss with the patient's doctor how to identify and treat them.

Nutrition

To manage HIV and AIDS, it is essential to rebuild and then maintain a proper nutritional status. Without adequate nutrition, the body cannot deal either with the disease or with its treatments.

AIDS patients sometimes fail to eat enough because their appetite is impaired. Chemical responses in the body can cause loss of appetite, nausea, and vomiting. Conditions such as thrush, esophagitis, or mouth sores may also make eating uncomfortable. In addition, some people with HIV have a condition known as malabsorption, which decreases the intestine's ability to absorb vital nutrients.

It is thought that HIV infection itself can impair intestinal function and absorption. Other opportunistic infections, although they do not affect the intestine directly, may alter the metabolism of iron, making less of it available for red blood cell production.

Because nutrition is crucial to continued health, dietary changes can be very effective. Insufficient levels of protein, fatty acids, and carnitine can contribute to muscle fatigue. Insufficient levels of vitamins B_{12}, A, and C; folate; carotene; and zinc are often associated with weight loss and fatigue. Work with an HIV-experienced nutritionist to develop a nutrition plan to help combat these deficiencies.

AIDS patients who continue to eat well tend to lose less weight and sometimes recover from opportunistic infections more completely. To learn more about the AIDS patient's nutritional needs, consult a physician who specializes in this field.

There are many strategies for dealing with appetite loss, nausea, vomiting, and diarrhea. In addition to giving the patient small, frequent meals, here are some other things you can do to control his digestive comfort.

For loss of appetite
Have the patient eat by a schedule. Give him foods that have lots of flavor (but don't add fat for flavor—use herbs and spices). Encourage him to eat with a friend, if possible, and to eat in a pleasant environment.

For nausea and vomiting
Have the patient replace lost fluids by drinking beverages between medications. Give him low-fat foods. Serve his food cold or at room temperature. Keep his upper body elevated after meals.

For diarrhea
Have the patient replace lost fluids. Give him low-fat foods. If the patient cannot tolerate milk, use lactose-free alternatives. Don't give the patient foods that contain crude fiber.

Fighting Fatigue

Many HIV and AIDS patients experience fatigue. It can take several forms:

- Physical fatigue is unusual tiredness after physical exertion.
- Mental fatigue is difficulty in focusing and concentration.
- Motivational fatigue is a lack of will or desire to engage in emotional, intellectual, or physical activities.

- Acute fatigue is generally short-lived, sudden in onset, and relieved by rest.
- Chronic fatigue lasts a long time, may be insidious in onset, and is usually not relieved by rest.

Although health care providers have come to understand the biology of HIV and AIDS much better over the years, some of them still dismiss these symptoms as being untreatable or even psychosomatic.

When a person becomes overly tired or anemic, the body tries to compensate in a number of ways. The heart rate increases, as does the respiratory rate. Certain capillary beds (tiny blood vessels in the tissues) open wider in an attempt to provide more oxygen to vital tissues, while other capillary beds get smaller in an attempt to preserve oxygen. This erratic redistribution of blood causes a pale complexion and a cold sensation in those with anemia. Ironically, more oxygen is provided to critical organs such as the heart and brain, and to muscles. This increased activity, however, produces an even greater need for oxygen, again, resulting in fatigue, weakness, palpitations, and shortness of breath as the body struggles to compensate.

Lifestyle and Fatigue

Exercise helps to reduce fatigue. The more carefully planned and regular it is, the better. An unfit person has less energy, and many studies have found that exercise is highly beneficial to people with HIV. The patient's exercise program should be individualized, based on her level of fitness and her age. Weight lifting builds up muscle tissue, where the protein required to make energy is stored, and aerobic exercise builds up heart function and increases oxygen intake.

Problems with sleeping at night can cause fatigue in the daytime. Some AIDS patients have trouble falling asleep, while others can fall asleep but wake up frequently. The caregiver should urge the patient to consider eliminating coffee, black tea, and cola drinks, all of which contain caffeine. Alcohol can also cause sleep disturbances and should be used in moderation, if at all.

Anxiety and depression are common among people with HIV and AIDS. The caregiver must be alert to the patient's radical mood swings. Encourage the patient to join a support group if possible. To locate the group nearest you, contact your local health authority or reference library.

Cancer

There are many types of cancer. The success of treatment depends primarily on what type of cancer the patient has, on his age, and on his strength and constitution.

The extreme conditions of cancer treatment generally require that the medical team and the family–caregiver team work together. The patient will often require a caregiver for the rest of his life.

Addressing the Physical Problems

Cancer and its treatments cause constant and ongoing discomfort. Common symptoms include nausea, fatigue, lack of appetite, pain caused by the disease itself, and sometimes pain caused by the treatment. Radiation therapy and chemotherapy have unpleasant side effects. Surgical procedures, such as colostomy or bone marrow transplant, are painful and debilitating.

The nausea that results from cancer treatment can be managed by medication. If the patient's nausea is not being managed adequately, you should urge her to discuss this issue with her physician.

Caregivers need to be especially sensitive to the degree of pain that the patient is experiencing. Some patients will be stoic even in the face of severe pain. Others, particularly the elderly, may give you confusing messages about it because they themselves may be suffering from dementia and memory loss. In all cases, pain can be significantly reduced with appropriate medication. Often morphine is prescribed for this purpose. Families and caregivers should be forceful with the medical staff in supporting a patient's right to have morphine if necessary. Physicians are sometimes reluctant to prescribe morphine, because strong doses may cause hallucinations. This is usually more uncomfortable for family members than it is for anyone else.

Finally, the cancer patient may be on a restricted or well-defined diet. It is essential that any dietary guidelines be followed. Maintaining proper nutritional status is crucial to recovery from cancer.

Addressing the Psychological Problems

The fear of an untimely death is often the first reaction of the person who is diagnosed with cancer. By the time the patient needs a caregiver, this fear may have moderated, but it is fantasy to believe that the patient is not afraid, no matter how brave she is. She may, of course, be concerned about other things as well and may even be obsessed with issues of personal comfort.

While both patient and caregiver should confront the reality of death, and may feel overwhelmed by the horror of the illness itself, it is crucial for the caregiver to remain optimistic, because fortunately some patients do recover.

Patients deal psychologically with cancer in many different ways. Some fight it with all their will. They seek help, change their lifestyles, and even actively take responsibility for the course of treatment. Some of these patients will be very angry, and their anger may fuel a determination not to die. The sensitive caregiver must be prepared for this and should even steel himself against possible abuse.

Some cancer patients go into denial. They are unable to accept the reality of their condition and act and talk as if nothing were wrong. Interestingly enough, deniers have the second-best survival rate, after those feisty, difficult people who oppose their doctors. So if the patient is a denier, the caregiver may do best just to play along.

Other patients become depressed and passive. They take no interest in their treatment, as if they have given up all hope of living.

Never forget that all cancer patients are confused and frightened about the future, so their emotions will generally be erratic. No matter what he says, the caregiver should readily accept the way the patient has chosen to deal with his disease. Your clear acceptance and sensitive support will make all the difference to him.

Depression, fear, anxiety, and complex psychological struggles are inherent in dealing with cancer. I believe that every patient should be encouraged to attend a cancer support group. These exist in every community and can often contribute significantly to the patient's well-being. Hospital social workers can put you in contact with local support groups. For more information, see the resources listed in appendix B.

In addition, cancer patients often confide in the caregiver herself. When this happens, you may learn about the patient's most intimate concerns. Sometimes the patient has become estranged from a family member, and you can act as mediator to bring them together. Or the patient may yearn to see some old friend, and you can act as messenger.

Alzheimer's Disease

Alzheimer's disease is a form of dementia that is characterized by disorientation to time and place and by loss of short-term memory. The signs and symptoms of Alzheimer's disease are caused by a breakdown in the neurotransmitters of the brain. It can be likened to a computer program when bits and pieces of information appear scrambled, then the system crashes.

The Alzheimer's patient may forget what year it is, what day it is, and where things are located in the house. He may forget how to read or write. He may have difficulty remembering the names of familiar people. To the caregiver, the patient may seem like an erratic amnesiac. As the disease progresses, the patient's speech becomes confused, degenerating eventually into meaningless sounds. In the end, he may no longer recognize the members of his own family.

Alzheimer's disease is an illness that severely tests the patience of everyone involved. In the early stages of Alzheimer's, the patient is frustrated, angry, and depressed as he becomes aware that he is losing his mental capacity.

The cause of Alzheimer's disease is unknown, and at present there is no known cure. Treatment remains problematic, although drugs can sometimes be prescribed that slow down the process of deterioration. Alzheimer's is usually diagnosed by eliminating all other possible causes for the patient's dementia. There is as yet no test that can provide a definitive diagnosis.

The single most important thing to do if you suspect that someone you know has Alzheimer's is to have an entire series of tests run on her by a qualified neurologist. The signs of many other conditions that can be successfully treated (drug interactions, brain tumors) resemble the signs of Alzheimer's disease.

The Challenge

When the patient has Alzheimer's, the caregiver's duties are not easy; they are time-consuming and challenging. This is especially true for family caregivers, who will experience anguish as they watch someone they love gradually losing her faculties.

You must help the patient with whatever activities she finds difficult or can no longer perform. These activities may range from doing housework to putting on her shoes.

It is important to protect the patient who is confused and incapacitated. You must make sure that her health needs are taken care of, even though she cannot describe to you how she feels. You may have to make all her social and medical appointments for her. You may have to keep her from wandering off and getting lost. You should make sure that she is able to sit and walk in a safe, secure environment, such as a fenced yard with soft grass and level paths. You may have to watch her as closely as you would a small child, so that she doesn't burn herself accidentally on a stove that she no longer recognizes as being hot.

An Alzheimer's caregiver has the creative challenge of helping the patient to stay occupied. He has lost many of his capacities and interests, but you can enhance his experiences by finding meaningful activities for him. Professionals in Alzheimer's care emphasize activities, such as looking at photo albums, that utilize the mental processes that the patient is losing—that is, his memory and his knowledge of time, place, and events. Family caregivers must carefully evaluate how realistic it is to stress demanding activities, even activities that were once familiar to the patient. It is important for all concerned not to add to the patient's stress level, which may already be high, and enable the person to experience success instead of constant failure.

It can be frustrating to communicate with Alzheimer's patients. Keep in mind that they are on a strange inner journey of resolution. They seek precision, focus, and clarity, although it may not seem as if they do. The caregiver must learn how to communicate with and relate to the patient without using words. This can be a real challenge, but communicating in this way can immediately establish a loving, caring relationship between you and the patient. Sitting quietly with him, giving him a hug or a shoulder rub, massaging his hands—all this communicates love and acceptance beyond words and may help to give the patient a sense of inner peace.

The family caregiver may find it difficult to engage in this kind of wordless communication. It is hard to see a person you know and love become so dependent and childlike. Yet who better to care for him than those who know him intimately and love him the most? Because you know him so well, you can "read" him better than anyone else. The very fact that you can do this may provide him with the comfort he so desperately needs.

Most people in the early stages of Alzheimer's are extremely angry, frustrated, and depressed, as I have already explained. The caregiver should check to see whether there is anything in the patient's immediate environment that may be adding to her stress. All too often, Alzheimer's patients are put on psychiatric medication without any attempt made to determine the cause of their anger.

Sensitive caregivers are often more aware of the patient's unspoken fears and anxieties when they recognize that Alzheimer's behavior usually serves a purpose. For example, Alzheimer's patients often engage in a great deal of agitated pacing, walking, and wandering. Sometimes the patient does this to calm his feelings of anxiety. Knowing this, the caregiver can facilitate the process.

Many Alzheimer's patients lose their sense of taste. This can cause them to stop eating, which may lead to malnutrition. The patient often compensates by raiding the refrigerator at night, usually eating something immediately gratifying, like ice cream. Sugar cravings are intense for people with dementia. It is important to intensify the flavors of the patient's food in order to maintain his interest in eating. A healthy way of doing this is by substituting herbs and spices for fatty condiments. By preparing good, wholesome meals and providing plenty of nutritious snacks, you can help to keep the patient well nourished.

Caring for the Caregiver

I recommend that anyone who is caring for an Alzheimer's patient attend one of the many caregiver support groups sponsored by the Alzheimer's Association. These meetings are superbly inform-ative. No one can fully predict all the challenges that may arise in caring for someone with this strange disease, but there is a strong chance that someone else has experienced something similar to what you are experiencing and has found a solution that will work for you.

Stroke

According to the American Medical Association, one-third of all peo-ple who have a stroke will die, one-third will suffer severe damage, and one-third will remain essentially unimpaired. It is the ones who suffer severe damage who are likely to need caregivers. Typically, a stroke will affect one side of the body more than the other. A really massive stroke, however, may affect both sides equally—with gen-eral paralysis. Even under the worst circumstances, a degree of recov-ery is possible, even in the elderly. This is why therapy for the stroke victim is of vital importance.

After a stroke, it is typical to have problems with comprehension, vision, verbalization, and movement. Since it takes a while for neural pathways to heal and reroute, there is often an interim period when the person finds it hard to think straight. Depending on the severity of the stroke, it may take some time for the patient to understand clearly what is going on or what is being said to him. The caregiver needs to be patient, optimistic, and encouraging during this period.

The patient may experience problems with her vision. She may see double or not see clearly. Depth of vision may also be disturbed, so the patient must take great care in climbing up stairs or stepping down. These problems will usually resolve over time, but obviously the patient must not drive until she can see normally again. It is also wise not to get a new prescription for eyeglasses, since the patient's vision will be changing soon. The caregiver should ask the patient's doctor when this stabilization is likely to occur.

The patient's speech is sometimes temporarily affected. Diction may become slurred and difficult to understand. It may be hard for the patient to find the right word. For example, the patient might think, "Where is the cat?" but actually say, "Where is the green?" He will know that "green" is the wrong word, but he will be unable to say "cat." This can be embarrassing and frustrating for both him and the caregiver. Both parties will need great patience and a sense of humor to sort these confusions out.

It can be very hard for the patient to move well, or even to move at all, after a stroke. Therapy helps, but so does willpower. To recover normal movement takes time, patience, self-discipline, and determination. The caregiver can encourage and cheer the person who is struggling to recover.

The patient may experience changes in bathroom habits. She may find that she needs to urinate or defecate more frequently. She may experience constipation, bowel infrequency, or urinary incontinence. These problems happen to almost half of all stroke victims, so the caregiver should reassure the patient that she is not alone and that these problems are nothing to be ashamed of. Special incontinence wear is readily available. Any nurse can help the patient to decide which type works best for her and is the most discreet and comfortable. Be certain that the patient protects her skin from chafing, redness, or heat rash, all of which can easily develop if she wears incontinence garments.

The incontinent patient's bed should be waterproofed with an appropriate protective covering. An inexpensive yet effective technique is to use heavy plastic garden bags. Place them underneath the sheets where the patient's lower body is likely to lie.

Even acts as simple as sitting centrally on a toilet seat may become more difficult after a stroke. The caregiver needs to guide the patient carefully under these delicate circumstances.

Changes in sexual abilities are also to be expected. The patient's sex drive will diminish following a stroke, but it is likely to return to its previous level over time, and the caregiver should encourage the patient not to worry about this.

Stroke patients may have difficulty chewing and swallowing. A doctor or physical therapist can suggest ways of dealing with this problem. If the stroke has damaged the patient's throat muscles, he may choke on thin liquids, such as fruit juices or even water. It may be necessary to thicken these drinks by adding gelatin or baby rice gruel (which is not as bad as it sounds). Sometimes drinking through a straw solves this problem.

Blood clots, especially in the legs, pose a risk to stroke patients. The doctor will be alert to this possibility. Meanwhile, caregivers must be alert for pain and swelling in the patient's legs, which could indicate the presence of a clot. If the patient experiences these symptoms, the doctor may suggest that he wear elastic support hose, known as antiembolism stockings, and that he keep his legs raised above heart level whenever he is resting.

Most stroke victims suffer from high blood pressure. They are often overweight and many of them smoke. It is important to encourage these patients to lose weight and to stop smoking. Caregivers can help by providing nutritious low-fat meals. They should also persuade the patient to join an antismoking program. There are many such programs to choose from. They are usually free and often incorporate effective methods, such as ear point acupuncture, to reduce the craving for nicotine. Homeopathic remedies have also been used for this purpose.

Time is the stroke victim's greatest friend. It is very important for the patient to accept that the healing process cannot be rushed. Relearning old skills takes time, and the patient must be willing to relax and concentrate on learning gradually.

Fear, anxiety, and depression often follow a stroke. It is frightening for the patient to lose so much physical control. He may feel that he will never again be the person that he once was. Caregivers need to be aware that this grief for the loss of a previous life is normal. At the same time, if it deepens into an emotional immobility, it becomes depression. That may be when medical intervention is necessary. Showing sympathy with the patient's change of perspective will help, especially if you let him know that his feelings are quite normal. However, it is also very important for the patient to practice positive thinking. The caregiver can encourage the patient to be optimistic by reminding him that seven out of ten stroke victims eventually recover well enough to live independently again. This is certainly a hopeful statistic.

Heart Disease

Heart problems are extremely common among people over fifty. People with high blood pressure or diabetes are at the greatest risk. There are several emergencies specific to heart patients. The two most common ones are angina and heart failure.

Angina is pain in the chest often following exertion or shock. It is the result of insufficient blood supply reaching the heart. Angina typically takes about fifteen minutes to subside. Speak calmly and reassuringly to the patient. If the patient is in pain, place a nitroglycerine tablet under his tongue, where it will dissolve. If the pain continues, give him another tablet after five minutes or so. If the pain is still present five minutes later, repeat the process. But if three tablets have no effect, call 911 or take the patient to the emergency room immediately.

Heart failure has many causes. It is most often characterized by labored breathing. When this occurs, the patient must sit up immediately. If shortness of breath continues, take the patient to the emergency room. If the problem recurs, the doctor may prescribe extra oxygen for use at home. In that case, you will need to learn how to operate the oxygen tank safely. The patient should also sleep in a semireclining bed with pillows piled high or in a raised-head hospital-style bed. This will enable him to breathe more easily.

Other signs and symptoms of heart failure include fatigue, a persistent cough, anxiety, shallow breathing, wheezing, rapid pulse, profuse perspiration, insomnia, and fluid retention. If the patient is retaining fluid, her legs or feet may swell, or she may gain weight suddenly. You should keep her as active as possible during the day.

Heart failure patients seldom recover. Usually, they gradually fade away until death finally comes to them.

A Word of Caution: Caregivers should be on the alert for the following symptoms of heart attack:

- Intermittent or continuous pressure in the chest area.
- Tightness or pain that starts in the chest and radiates to the shoulders, arms, and neck. In women, this may be a pressure or tingling feeling anywhere above the waist.
- Shortness of breath, nausea, vomiting, sweating, dizziness, or fainting.

If the patient is experiencing the symptoms of a heart attack, encourage him to lie down and loosen his clothing. Then call 911, or rush the patient to the nearest emergency room.

CHAPTER 3

Professional Resources

The Doctor

If you are a caregiver responsible for someone who is ill or disabled, the most important professional person in your life is the patient's medical doctor. Your choice of a physician will reflect the quality of care that the patient receives.

Ask yourself the following questions when deciding whether a certain doctor is the right one for you and your patient:

- Do you like this doctor intuitively? Do you feel that you and he can communicate well with each other?
- Does this doctor respect your opinions and your needs?
- Is this doctor readily available in an emergency, or is it difficult to get an appointment to see her?
- Does this doctor provide help in contacting other professional resources? Does he offer this help willingly, even if you want a second opinion?

- Do you have confidence that this doctor could handle the patient's dying process well? Could she provide you and the patient with help and support?

You need a doctor who will make you feel secure. If yours does not, you should probably find another doctor.

When visiting the patient's doctor, it is very important to get clear in your own mind what you need. Write down everything you want to talk about and bring a list of all the medications the patient is taking when you go to the office. Remember to make notes of all required medications.

You should also familiarize yourself with the patient's insurance and with Medicaid or Medicare, if applicable. Make sure that you know what each will pay for, and under what conditions. For example, some insurance plans will pay for certain things (even a hospital bed for home use) only if the doctor provides a written order. There are many things you can get in the way of equipment and services, but your patient's doctor may not think of everything unless you know exactly what you need. So ask as many questions as you can, no matter how foolish you may think they are.

Sometimes the patient's doctor may not see the point of certain services. In chapter 1, I described how when a ninety-seven year-old woman had a stroke, her doctor made no provision for her to get rehabilitation services. Her family researched what services were available and found the appropriate help. The old woman was able to resume a more active life until her death the following year. No one is ever so old that learning to live independently is a waste of time.

Make good use of the doctor's nurses and office staff. They can often provide you with a wealth of information, and they know the system. They have seen a lot of people deal with a lot of different situations, and they may have helpful suggestions for you. The nurses and staff can also act as a diplomatic bridge between you and the doctor.

HMOs and Hospitals

HMO stands for health maintenance organization. Although the HMO system is much criticized, it offers several advantages. People in the doctor–HMO partnership are usually very familiar with the resources available in the community and can easily make appropriate referrals. In an HMO there is usually at least one person—generally a social worker—who is aware of all these resources and can help you make use of them. This health professional can tell you how to get the services you need and even how to pay for them. You may need to be persistent to get an appointment, but once there, you should ask this person a lot of questions. You will usually find that there is a great deal of help to be had by asking.

In larger HMOs, such as Kaiser Permanente, there are a variety of specialists who can help you in many other ways. They can provide information about everything from how to obtain home sickroom equipment to how to apply for Medicaid.

Shortcomings of HMOs

One disadvantage of HMOs is that they pressure doctors to always consider the cost of the choices that they make. This can mean that those choices are not always the best ones for the patient.

Some HMO doctors even subtly discourage patients from seeking a second opinion. This is another reason why you need to know as much as possible about the patient's condition. Research the ways in which it is usually treated. The days of being a passive receptor are over.

Hospital Health Professionals

Hospitals also employ specialists in a variety of areas: medical, financial, rehabilitation, and so on. And like HMOs, they provide a social worker who should be able to help you to get any information that you need. This social worker will know what special services are available through the hospital, including patient support groups, caregiver support groups, and home health services.

Social workers are also familiar with special financial programs that might help you or the patient. There are special aid programs for refugees, pregnant women, cancer patients, indigent Parkinson's patients, and many others.

Hospital staff can put you in contact with agencies that provide help when the patient comes home: home health aides, visiting nurses, and Meals on Wheels. The last provides nutritionally balanced meals at little or no cost. Meals on Wheels can help overcome the problem of poor nutrition, which I believe is what causes many old people to need care in the first place.

Pharmacists

One person often overlooked as a source of information and help is the pharmacist. Most people go to the pharmacy just to pick up their prescription and pay the bill. These people are missing an opportunity for consultation. The pharmacist is a highly trained professional who often knows more about the side effects and interactions of drugs than the physician does. If the patient is taking a combination of drugs, the pharmacist's familiarity with her case could prove invaluable in preventing unforeseen complications. The pharmacist can also advise you on appropriate generic substitutes for brand-name prescriptions, which can save you a lot of money.

So next time you go in to pick up a prescription, engage in an honest dialogue with the pharmacist. You'll be glad you did.

Home Health Services

Home health agencies deliver health care to a patient in his own home. Their services may enable the patient to remain at home, thus delaying or completely avoiding a move to an assisted-living facility or nursing home.

Nurses, therapists, social workers, and nutritionists are employed by home health agencies to deliver the skilled care that the patient's physician prescribes. Home health aides and homemaker assistants can help the patient with daily activities, personal care, and housework. Some agencies also provide medical supplies and equipment.

Registered nurses (RNs) perform skilled tasks, such as giving injections, drawing blood, taking blood pressure, caring for wounds, and inserting catheters. They monitor medications and teach family members how to perform any special procedures that may be necessary. RNs work closely with the doctor and pharmacist.

A physician may prescribe home visits by a registered nurse if the patient is returning from a hospital stay involving surgery. The RN will generally continue these home visits until the patient is healed.

Social workers provide short-term counseling and arrange other community services to help families resolve physical, emotional, and financial problems.

Nutritionists plan special diets. They also teach family members the importance of following a prescribed nutritional plan—not just for the patient but for themselves.

Therapists perform physical, speech, respiratory, and occupational therapies in the home.

Visits from home health aides are always helpful. These aides can assist the physically impaired with bathing, household chores, cooking meals, cleaning, doing the laundry, shopping, and running errands. Physicians do not generally refer home health aides.

Many home care agencies charge fees according to a sliding scale based on income. This is especially true of nonprofit agencies and agencies that are affiliated with local government. Some senior services, or your local Area Agency on Aging, also offer these services. Medicare will sometimes reimburse expenses for such care.

Finding conscientious help to come into your home and share the responsibility of caring for a family member is a challenge. Allowing a stranger into your private life may also be intimidating. It is always best first to consider getting help from a family member or a friend in whom you have confidence.

If you hire a caregiver from an agency, it will already have checked the person's background, including references from previous employers and any possible criminal record. If you need to seek out a professional caregiver with specialized nursing skills, the visiting nurse program in your community can help.

If you hire a person directly (by running an ad in a newspaper, for example), you will have to perform a background check yourself. This is important. I cannot emphasize strongly enough that you should telephone several of the person's former employers. (Personal references may not be as reliable.) Ask them how reliable, helpful, and honest this person was. For more about hiring a caregiver, see the checklists on pages 61 and 62.

There are also consultants called private care managers (sometimes professional social workers) who offer specialized, comprehensive care planning and coordinating to families of patients who need extensive home care. They will help you to define the patient's care needs by making both immediate and long-range plans. In addition, they will locate a home care worker, locate all health services, and manage finances or find a professional who will. They will make contact with a transportation service, take the patient to the doctor, or make sure that hot meals are delivered to the home.

These care managers can be expensive, but I believe that they can make all the difference if you suddenly find yourself caring for a seriously disabled patient and have no idea how to do it.

Hospice

Hospice care (also known as palliative care) is appropriate when the goal shifts from active treatment and cure to comfort and relief of suffering in a dying patient.

Hospice treatment is based on continuity of care. Care can be provided in the hospital or in a palliative care unit as the need arises. Inpatient hospice units also exist, although there are not very many of them in the United States at present.

For the most part, however, hospice care is provided in the home. Twenty-four-hour help is available by telephone seven days a week for the families of patients receiving hospice home care.

Many people experience hospice home care as comforting and less isolating than hospital end-of-life care. The patient can remain involved in many aspects of family life, and the family experiences less disruption. Hospice home care is covered by Medicare for patients who are disabled or are sixty-five or older.

Getting the Best from Hospice

In order to be sure you are getting the best hospice care,

- You need to be clear about your needs.
- You need to learn the options.
- You need to ask questions and pursue leads until you obtain the kinds of services you want.

This may require tenacity, but there are many people who are willing to help you and your loved one.

Mental Health Services

It is not uncommon for older adults to experience depression or emotional and behavioral problems. Alcohol and drug dependency are also common in this population. The people most often sent for shock treatment for depression (yes, this practice is still used!) are widowed women over age sixty-five. And the biggest group of drug addicts among elders in this country are older adults who have become addicted to doctor-prescribed medications, such as sleeping pills, Valium, and barbiturates.

When the patient shows signs of mental illness or addiction, finding help can be difficult, especially in rural areas and small towns. You need to identify the outpatient and inpatient psychiatric facilities, community mental health centers, and private practitioners in your area.

When considering mental health treatment, ask the following questions.

Where Is the Service Delivered?

Mental health services can be found in inpatient and outpatient hospital settings, private offices, nursing homes, and private homes.

Is the Service Covered by the Patient's Insurance?

Be sure to ask whether the service is covered by the patient's HMO, Medicare, preferred provider organization (PPO), private insurance, or managed care plan.

Review the patient's policies and benefits to determine the limits of coverage before beginning treatment. Be aware that some providers will offer a reduced or sliding fee scale if the patient cannot pay the full amount.

Do You Qualify for Government Benefits?

You or the patient may qualify for federal, state, or local benefit programs. Inquire at your state's Health and Human Services, Mental Health and Mental Retardation (MHMR), and Medicaid offices. (The caregiver may qualify because of caring for the patient.)

Local county and city offices can also direct you to programs for which you or the patient may be eligible. Understand that Medicare provides only limited mental health benefits.

Hiring a Professional Caregiver

Sometimes it's necessary to hire a professional caregiver. Here are some questions to ask and points to consider.

About the Agency

- What services are provided?
- What is the cost? Does the agency accept Medicare and Medicaid?
- Are the workers certified?
- How are the workers supervised?
- How is the plan of care determined?
- Is someone available twenty-four hours a day in case of emergency?
- Is the agency licensed or accredited?
- Can the agency provide references?
- Are the workers trained to meet the needs of patients with Parkinson's, Alzheimer's, and so forth?
- How often do the workers take continuing education courses?

About the Individual Caregiver

- Is the candidate certified in any way?
- What experience and training does the candidate have?
- Is the candidate respectful and well groomed?
- Does the patient respond well to the candidate?
- What duties will the candidate be expected to perform? Does the candidate agree to perform them?
- Is the candidate readily available when needed?
- Does the candidate have professional references from former employers?

Choosing a Nursing Home

Sometimes the appropriate choice is long-term care outside the home. In choosing a nursing facility, ask the following questions.

Licensing and Certification

- Does the facility have a framed, posted license from the state Department of Health?
- Does the administrator have a current license from the state Board of Examiners for Nursing Home Administrators?
- Is the facility certified to participate in Medicare or Medicaid or both?

Location

- Is the facility conveniently located for the patient's personal doctor?
- Is it conveniently located for frequent visits by the patient's family and friends?

Accident Prevention

- Are the rooms and halls well lit and free from glare?
- Are the rooms free of hazards underfoot?

- Are the chairs sturdy and not easily tipped over?
- Is there a nonslip surface on the hallway and bathroom floors?
- Are there handrails in the hallways and grab bars in the bathroom?

Fire Safety

- Does the facility have a sprinkler system?
- Does the facility have smoke detectors?
- Are written emergency evacuation plans posted?
- Are fire drills held regularly?
- Are exit doors clearly marked, unlocked, and unobstructed?
- Are stairways enclosed? Are the doors to stairways kept closed?

Bedrooms

- Do bedrooms open into the hall?
- Is there a window in each bedroom?
- Are there no more than four beds per room?
- Is there easy access to each bed?
- Does each bed have curtains?
- Is there a nurse call bell by each bed?
- Is there fresh drinking water by each bed?
- Is there at least one comfortable chair per patient?
- Are there enough reading lights?
- Are there plenty of clothes closets and drawers?
- Is there room for a wheelchair to maneuver?
- Is the room and facility air-conditioned?

Toilet and Bathing Facilities

- Is the toilet located in a room that is easy for a wheelchair patient to use?

- Is there a sink in this room?
- Is there a nurse call bell?
- Are there handgrips on or near toilets?
- Do the bathtubs and showers have nonslip surfaces?
- Is the bathroom well lit?

Cleanliness

- Is the facility free of unpleasant odors?
- Are incontinent patients given prompt attention?
- Does the facility seem to be in good repair?

Day Room

- Do the residents appear to be using the day room?
- Does it have lamps, tables, and comfortable chairs?
- Are books and games available?

Dining Room and Food Services

- Is the dining room attractive and pleasant?
- Does it have comfortable chairs and tables?
- Do the meals match the posted menu? Are they attractively served?
- Do residents who need help with eating receive it?
- Are meals served on a regular schedule?
- Are residents encouraged to eat in the dining room?
- Are special diets available?

Kitchen

- Are the food preparation, dishwashing, and garbage areas separated?
- Is the food that needs refrigeration not left standing on counters?
- Do the kitchen help observe sanitation rules?

Isolation Room

- Is there at least one bed and bedroom available for patients with contagious illnesses?

Grounds

- Is there an outdoor area where residents can sit or walk?
- Is there a secure outdoor area for residents with dementia?
- Are the grounds attractive, well kept, and accessible to residents?

Medical Services

- Is a physician available in case of emergency?
- Do the patients have access to regular medical attention at all times?
- Do patients receive a thorough physical immediately before or upon admission?
- Are medical records and plan of care kept secure?
- Are other medical services, such as dentists and optometrists, available regularly?
- Do residents have the freedom to choose their own pharmacy?
- Is emergency transportation available?

Nursing Services

- In a skilled nursing facility, or a nursing facility with twenty-five or more beds, is the nursing staff overseen by a registered nurse?
- Is there a licensed practical nurse or an RN on all shifts seven days per week?
- Are nurse's aides certified through a state-approved training program?

Activities Program

- Can residents participate in activities that they choose?
- Are there group and individual activities?
- Are residents encouraged but not forced to participate?
- Are there outside trips for those who can go on them?
- Do volunteers from the community work with residents?
- Is there an activities director or coordinator on the staff?
- Are activities offered to residents who are confined to their beds or rooms?

Religious Observances

- Are arrangements made for residents to worship as they please?
- Are religious observances a matter of choice?

Social Services

- Is a social worker available to help residents and their families?
- Are family forums held on a regular basis?
- Does the facility have a residents' council that meets on a regular basis?
- Does the facility have a family council that meets on a regular basis?

Grooming

- Are barbers available for men? Are hairdressers and beauticians available for women?

Laundry

- Is personal clothing laundered in the facility?
- Are special efforts made to prevent loss of clothing?
- Is the cost of laundry included in the monthly fee?

Special Considerations

- Does the facility provide physical, speech, and occupational therapies to meet the residents' needs?
- Can arrangements be made to meet other special needs of the residents?
- Is additional supervision or assistance available for confused residents or those with dementia?
- Are orientation clues, such as directional signs and large clocks, conspicuously displayed?

Staff

- Is the staff courteous and helpful to residents and their families?
- Is the administrator available to residents and their families during normal business hours?

Financial Considerations

- Does the contract clearly state what services and goods are and are not included in the basic fee? Do the goods and services listed include personal toiletries, diapers, special diets, therapies, medical supplies, and extra supervision or assistance?
- Are the monthly charges prorated in case the resident is discharged or dies before the end of the billing period?
- Are residents given a monthly itemized accounting of services and fees and an accounting of their personal funds available?

Residents' Rights

- Are the residents informed of their rights and responsibilities?
- Are they encouraged to exercise their rights as citizens, such as their right to vote?

- Are residents encouraged to manage their own finances? If not, do they receive an accounting of their pocket or personal money from the facility or guardian?
- Are residents given privacy for telephone calls and visits?
- Can residents choose their own physician, pharmacy, and care providers as long as they can afford the fees?
- Are they encouraged to take part in planning their own care?
- May they keep their own clothes and possessions, given space limitations?
- Are married couples encouraged to share a room if they want to?
- Are important legal telephone numbers posted? Do they include the numbers of the state Department of Health, the state Long-Term Care Ombudsman Program, and the Medicaid Fraud Control unit?
- Is there an admission preference given due to the source of the payment?
- Were you given information on the facility's waiting list, including the number of people on the list and the dates when those people were placed on the list?
- Do residents appear alert, well dressed, and well cared for?
- Are visiting hours convenient for family and friends?
- Is the overall atmosphere clean, comfortable, and secure?

CHAPTER 4

Paying for Health Care

Nothing is more worrisome than trying to figure out how to pay for the needs of a person who requires long-term care. How will this person be taken care of if the family can no longer manage?

Everyone has heard tales of families spending almost all their resources on long-term care. Only a few years ago, some spouses actually felt they had to divorce each other in order for one of them to get the care he needed.

The United States desperately needs a health plan for all its citizens. It is the only developed country in the world that doesn't have one. Meanwhile, everyone who does have health coverage—and forty million Americans do not—must know how to get the care they need without bankrupting their entire families.

With health care, as with many things, the very rich and the very poor have, in some ways, the least to worry about. The rich can afford to pay for their care, and care of the very poor is mandated by federal law. Most people, however, fall somewhere in between these two extremes. This chapter tells you what you need to know in order to plan how to pay for the patient's medical care and services.

Entitlement Programs

The patient's illness, and its treatment, can interfere with his ability to work, and this may cause financial difficulties for the entire family. The good news is that many government programs, called entitlements, are designed to help people in this situation.

The patient has earned the right to these benefits through his tax contributions. The common stumbling block for obtaining help from entitlements is the misconception that one hasn't really earned this help—that it's a handout. The truth is that the patient or her family members have been paying all along for the possibility that she might someday need to benefit from these programs.

Entitlements are available on the federal, state, and local levels. Eligibility guidelines vary from state to state. To learn what the patient is eligible to receive, contact your local Social Security Administration (SSA) office, your local Department of Public Welfare, and your hospital social worker.

Following are brief descriptions of the most important entitlement programs.

Social Security pays monthly retirement, disability, and survivor benefits for insured workers and their dependents. Eligibility is based on number of years of employment in Federal Insurance Contributions Act–taxed jobs, together either with age or with a disabling condition that is expected to continue for at least one year and that renders the worker unable to engage in gainful employment. (Gainful employment is defined as employment that pays at least five hundred dollars per month.) Eligibility is not based on assets or unearned income. Applications are processed through your local SSA office. Call 1-800-SSA-1213 to start the process.

Supplemental Security Income (SSI) is a monthly cash benefit available to low-income individuals. Applicants must be aged sixty-five or older, or blind or disabled. This benefit is based not on work history, but on current low income and asset status. Eligibility guidelines vary from state to state. Applicants may also qualify for Medicaid and food stamps. SSI is administered through Social Security.

Veterans Benefits offer pensions for low-income and disabled veterans. Health care is provided through VA facilities for vocational rehabilitation, disability, and even burial. Dependents and survivors may also be eligible for benefits. Apply through your local Department of Veterans Affairs.

It generally takes several months for applications to be approved. In the meantime, state disability programs can help to replace some of the patient's lost income. These state programs are administered locally through Workers' Compensation boards. The patient may also qualify for unemployment insurance if he is not disabled. Your local Department of Social Services may also manage federal block grants that provide public assistance cash benefits for low-income applicants.

COBRA is a federal act that allows individuals who lose employer health insurance coverage to buy group insurance for themselves and their families for a limited period of time. This may be helpful, especially through the waiting period before Medicare or Medicaid kicks in. To apply, contact the patient's employer or her group health insurance plan.

The Hill-Burton program provides some hospitals with federal funding to help eligible patients obtain treatments they might not otherwise be able to afford. Call 1-800-638-0742 for a list of participating hospitals in your area.

In the private sector, some pharmaceutical companies provide financial assistance with the cost of covered drugs for low-income patients. For a list of Pharmaceutical Indigent programs, call 1-800-762-4636. Many states offer senior prescription plans that provide low-cost medications for seniors. Contact your state Department of Aging for information.

Food stamps are coupons used for buying food. To be eligible for food stamps, the patient only has to be poor. Apply at your local Department of Social Services.

Finally, the Home Energy Assistance Program (HEAP) and the Weatherization Referral and Packaging Program (WRAP) help low-income homeowners and renters to pay for fuel and utilities or help them to weatherize their homes. Contact your local Department of Social Services, your local SSA office, or your hospital social worker to learn more about these programs.

Medicare

Medicare is the national health insurance program for people aged sixty-five and older. Generally, any elderly adult who is a citizen or permanent resident of the United States and who receives retirement benefits from Social Security or the Railroad Retirement Board is eligible for Medicare. Spouses of eligible people are also eligible if they are aged sixty-five or otherwise qualify.

Medicare has two parts. The first part covers hospital insurance, care in a nursing facility, home health, and hospice care. The second part covers medical insurance, doctor fees, outpatient hospital care, and other services.

Medicare also covers some nursing home or long-term care expenses. To qualify for Medicare nursing home benefits, the person must have been an inpatient at a hospital for at least three days and must have been discharged for no more than thirty days. Moreover, a physician must certify that the person requires skilled nursing care or rehabilitation that can be provided only in such a facility. If the patient qualifies, Medicare pays 100 percent of the costs for the first twenty days. From day twenty-one to day one hundred, the patient pays ninety-five dollars per day, and Medicare covers the difference. (This copayment can be handled by the patient's supplementary insurance, or by Medicaid if he has no insurance.) After day one hundred, Medicare ceases to pay anything.

This program is ideal, for example, for a patient who has fractured a hip or has had a stroke and who requires help with all activities as well as therapy on a daily basis, but who will not require help indefinitely. Medicare does not cover custodial care. Other services and products not covered by Medicare include: routine physicals, most dental care, dentures, routine foot care, hearing aids, eyeglasses, and outpatient prescription drugs.

Medigap

Medigap is specifically designed by Medicare law to supplement certain benefit gaps, such as deductibles and copayments. However, most of the medical services and products not covered by Medicare are not covered by Medigap either.

With respect to nursing home expenses, Medigap insurance may supplement Medicare benefits by covering the ninety-five-dollar copayment for the twenty-first through one hundredth day. So with a Medicare and a Medigap policy working jointly, long-term care benefits may be covered up to a maximum of one hundred days.

Medicare law defines ten standard Medigap benefit plans. Each plan offers a different combination of benefits and can be purchased in most states. The features of the individual policies will vary, however, from state to state.

Medicare HMO

A Medicare HMO is a managed care plan contracted with Medicare to provide all of Medicare's benefits to its members. It also provides most of the typical Medigap policy benefits, as well as prescription drugs, hearing aids, eye exams, routine physicals, hearing aids, and scheduled inoculations. For the first one hundred days of nursing home care, a Medicare HMO covers the full cost.

The HMO collects monthly premium payments from members and also from Medicare. But be careful. Should a member choose, without approval by the HMO, to receive services from a provider who is not part of the HMO network, the HMO either will not pay for the service or will pay for it at a reduced rate.

HMO coverage is more complex than the coverage provided by Medicare and a Medigap policy because each HMO has different regulations. Furthermore, if members move from one area to another, they may lose benefits or have them reduced. For more about choosing the best HMO, see "Tips for Choosing an HMO or a Managed Health Care Plan" later in this chapter.

Supplemental Coverage

Health care discount plans have become widely accepted as a means to help pay for some of these services and products not covered by Medicare. Some of these plans are excellent and very affordable.

A health care discount plan is not really an insurance plan. Members buy into the plan with a reasonably small monthly fee and receive a discount of up to 50 percent on goods and services not covered by Medicare. These might include prescription drugs, dental care, vision care, or hearing aids. The cost of these plans is modest—from nine to thirty dollars per month, depending on the discounts.

If you're interested in joining one of these plans, look at your Medicare coverage and Medigap policy to see what expenses are not covered. Then compare this list against the discounts the health care plan provides. (Caregivers often buy insurance, especially if dementia in the patient is suspected.) Do some comparison shopping; call a pharmacy that is affiliated with one of these plans and check their prices against what you usually pay. Anyone is eligible to participate in these discount plans. You just sign up and pay the monthly fee.

Medicaid

Medicaid may cover the patient's medical expenses with the help of Medicare, provided that the patient is over sixty-five and has a very low income. Medicaid is not health care insurance. It is a national, but state-operated, program designed to help low-income adults and children to pay their medical bills. To be eligible for federal funds, states have to provide Medicaid coverage for certain mandatory eligibility groups.

Medicaid is a safety net. If the patient has Medicare but cannot afford any other kind of insurance, Medicaid acts as secondary insurance and will help pay for things not covered by Medicare. Examples of things that Medicaid will pay for include doctor's care, limited prescription medicine, long-term care in a nursing home, hospital costs, eyeglasses, hearing aids, and family planning.

Over and above the federally mandated Medicaid benefits, each state elects the benefits that it will provide under Medicaid. Some states are now providing Medicaid assistance for long-term care in assisted living facilities. Each state determines the criteria for receiving these benefits. Eligibility is generally based on monthly income plus assets.

Many people do not realize that Medicaid provides personal care services to patients who are living at home. It does so in recognition of the fact that home care often makes the best economic sense for people who need long-term care. Personal care services provide assistance with activities of daily living, such as eating, bathing, dressing, personal hygiene, bladder and bowel elimination, and taking medications. These services must be:

- Authorized by a physician in accordance with a plan of treatment, or otherwise authorized in accordance with a service plan approved by the state.
- Provided by a qualified individual who is not a member of the patient's family.
- Furnished in a home or other location.

To receive these services, the patient must not be a hospital inpatient or a resident of a nursing facility, an intermediate care facility for the mentally retarded, or an institution for the treatment of mental disease.

Home- and Community-Based Waivers

Home- and community-based waivers may allow you to keep the patient at home and get Medicaid to pay for home helpers. It can be done.

The waiver program recognizes that many individuals at risk of institutionalization can and should be cared for in their homes to preserve their independence and their ties to their family. Home care costs less than institutional care, and of course, it is much more supportive as well.

The waiver program affords states the flexibility to develop and implement creative alternatives to institutionalizing Medicaid-eligible patients. It enables states to request waivers of certain federal rules that would otherwise limit treatment alternatives. It allows states to make home- and community-based services available to individuals who would otherwise qualify for Medicaid only if they were in an institutional setting.

The Social Security Act specifies seven services that may be utilized under the waiver program. They are case management, homemaker services, home health aide services, personal care services, adult day health, rehabilitation, and respite care. Other services, such as transportation, in-home support, meals, special communication, minor home modifications, and adult day care, may be provided subject to approval.

States have the flexibility to design each waiver program to best meet the needs of the populations they serve. Waiver services may be provided statewide, or they may be limited to specific geographic areas. They are provided to the elderly, the physically disabled, and the mentally ill. Waivers are also targeted to technology-dependent children and to individuals with AIDS. Check with your state regarding any of these services that you think your patient may be eligible to receive.

Navigating the System

I believe that every consumer needs to know the ins and outs of using the system to obtain the maximum benefits. All government bureaucracy is difficult to deal with, especially when it comes to paying out money. The key to getting the government to help pay for your medical care is to keep everything the law allows you to keep. Never spend money that you don't have to spend.

The Transfer of Assets

The patient is eligible to receive Medicaid only if she has very limited assets, as I have explained. However, it is possible to get around this limitation by transferring the patient's assets to another party before the Medicaid period begins.

Current law says that Medicaid can look back at all transfers of assets for the last thirty-six months. In some instances, regarding trusts, Medicaid may look back sixty months. If the transfer is made within these time limits, it will affect the eligibility of either the patient or her spouse to collect Medicaid payments for care. Furthermore, a person in a nursing home (or receiving equivalent services in a hospital) is ineligible for Medicaid coverage for a period of time after a gift or transfer of assets, whether by the person himself or by his spouse. For all these reasons, it is important to plan well ahead. No transfer of assets should be embarked on without first consulting an attorney.

Under the transfer rules, certain assets are exempt. For example, the patient's home is exempt if it is transferred to a spouse, a minor, a blind or disabled child of the patient who is receiving Medicaid for long-term care, a brother or sister of the patient who has equity interest in the home, or a son or daughter who resided in the home and provided care for at least two years to prevent the patient from being institutionalized.

Even when they are exempt, transfers between husband and wife should take place before the sick spouse goes on Medicaid. It is possible, however, for these transfers to be made after a Medicaid application has been filed and even after a decision on eligibility has been made.

Unmarried couples with jointly held assets or property should consult an attorney concerning the transfer of assets.

Excess Income Program

Another helpful provision of Medicare is the Excess Income program. This program allows families to become eligible for Medicaid even if their income exceeds the mandated limits. This is done by spending down to Medicaid levels during a three-month period. In some states, the Medicaid Excess Income program is available for persons who are over sixty-five or who are blind or disabled. If their income it too high to qualify for public assistance or SSI, but they spend down the excess on medical costs until they reach the Medicaid income level, they become eligible. The Excess Income program is not available in all states.

Spousal Impoverishment

Finally, the law specifies that the spouse of a nursing home patient may retain certain assets without affecting the patient's Medicaid eligibility. The exact amounts vary from state to state, but in general, the spouse can keep the house, the car, material goods, a lump sum of up to $80,000 (typically about $60,000), and a monthly income of about $1,200. (Note that income in the name of one spouse is considered available only to the spouse whose name it is in. Thus the income of the patient's spouse is not considered to be available to the institutionalized patient. If, however, the spouse has more than $2,019 in income per month, Medicaid will suggest that she contribute 25 percent of the excess over $201 to the institutionalized patient's medical care.)

In considering these and other factors, keep abreast of the Medicaid rules in your own state as well as the federal rules regarding assets and income. When you actually begin to plan, you would be wise to consult an attorney who specializes in elder law.

Other Ways to Protect Private Assets

In addition to the strategies outlined above, there are various other ways of protecting private assets. What follows is not intended to be legal advice. It is merely a description of courses of action that are commonly available. To find out what you should do, you must consult a lawyer who is experienced in elder law. There are some legal things that the patient's relatives can do, but protecting assets from the government is not one of them.

The patient or his relatives may want to consider one or more of these strategies:

- Move money into exempt assets. This means paying off a mortgage, car payments, and all debts.
- Set up a specialized trust through a good estate attorney. Possibilities include a family asset protection trust, an irrevocable asset protection trust, a testamentary trust, and a special needs trust.
- Set up a revocable living trust and joint ownership to protect retained assets.

More aggressive strategies include the following:

- Refuse to make assets available to a spouse in a nursing home. Unlikely as it may seem, relatives can refuse to augment Medicaid payments and nothing will happen to them.
- Set up a limited liability company or a family limited partnership to protect assets.
- Get a divorce.

Tips for Choosing an HMO or a Managed Health Care Plan

To evaluate an HMO or managed care plan, start with the summary of benefits, which is usually found in the company's promotional literature.

If you have a question about coverage, ask a representative of the company to get the information. If you can't get an important piece of information in writing, don't join the plan. Look at each of the following factors.

Choice of Doctors and Other Providers

Are the doctors, hospital, and other providers you already use included in the plan's network of providers? If they are, the tight restrictions of HMOs may not have much effect on you. If not, you may have to find new doctors, or use a hospital farther from your home. With PPOs, or HMOs with a point-of-service option, you may be allowed to use providers who are not in the network, but you will have to make a higher copayment when you do so.

Access to Specialists and Preventive Care

Can you easily get a referral to a specialist? Most plans require that the patient see her primary care physician first and get a referral to a specialist from him.

Total Cost

Add up the premiums and the other costs, especially copayments for physician visits and prescription drugs. See which plan is the least expensive, but remember that low premiums are only one factor to consider in choosing a plan.

Review Process

About 30 percent of Medicare managed care patients report having been denied coverage for treatments that their plans deemed to be medically unnecessary or experimental. If the patient is denied coverage for a treatment or service, Medicare will not help you if you decide to appeal. The review process is run by the plan. You will find the details explained in the summary of benefits booklet. Study them carefully for material for your appeal.

Extent of Service Area

Consider the extent of a plan's service area. If the service area is not broad enough to include a good selection of specialists, the patient may find her care choices limited. Also, see if the plan has extended service areas. Some plans permit you to arrange medical care away from home if you travel frequently.

Other Benefits

Some plans offer a variety of other features beyond basic Medicare coverage. These can include short-term custodial care, medical equipment, chiropractic care, acupuncture, acupressure, routine physical exams, foreign travel immunizations and emergency coverage, eye examinations and eyeglasses, hearing tests and hearing aids, dental work, after-hours advice and treatment, chronic disease management, and wellness programs.

Private Insurance

Private insurance can help pay the costs of medical and long-term expenses not covered by Medicare or Medicaid. But insurance plans are very specific about what they will and will not pay for. You need to know how to make your way through the maze.

If you want to get the most from private insurance, study the policy carefully. Talk to someone at the company but don't count on that person to tell you what you really need to know. An insurance company's goal is to make money. For unbiased advice, talk to the staff in your health care provider's office. Ask for their input.

You would also be wise to consult the local branch of the American Association of Retired Persons (AARP). They will probably have an insurance expert to help you. Unfortunately, many so-called long-term care insurance policies turn out to be useless when they are really needed. You sometimes find that the considerable monthly premiums do not cover care for Alzheimer's disease or other conditions.

Long-term care is the everyday help that the patient needs when illness or disability makes him unable to care for himself for a lengthy period of time. It can be provided at a nursing facility or assisted living facility. It can also be provided at home, with certified nurse's aides and licensed nurses. Long-term care insurance helps to pay for this. Bear in mind that the average cost of nursing home care is now estimated to be between $36,000 and $50,000 a year. The average length of stay is three years.

Obviously, buying long-term care insurance makes sense—or does it? The United Seniors Health Cooperative suggests that most people cannot afford long-term care insurance unless:

- The patient has more than $75,000 in assets, excluding the value of his home, for each person in his household.

- The patient has an annual retirement income of over $30,000 per person in the household and can comfortably afford the policy premiums.
- The patient has heart problems, rheumatoid arthritis, Alzheimer's, Parkinson's, emphysema, or some other chronic condition. (These conditions are not necessarily affordable, but insurance would be helpful in the costs of treatments.)

I suggest that you carefully study the family health profile to decide whether long-term care insurance is worth purchasing. Premiums exceeding 5 to 7 percent of one's annual income may simply make the policy unaffordable. If one cannot afford the premiums during the several years when one may actually need the care, then the situation demands another solution. If one can afford long-term care insurance, look at lifestyle, family history, life expectancy, and current health status. If the risks seem to be high and the patient is not already suffering from a chronic medical condition, long-term care insurance may be the right choice for that individual. Note also that if one is female, single, or widowed, the chances of needing long-term care are greater because women are more likely to live longer.

If one chooses to get long-term care insurance, start by examining a few different policies. Pay special attention to the premiums, the benefits, the benefit triggers, and the limitations. Investigate whether benefits are paid only for nursing home stays, or whether they are also paid for stays at assisted living facilities and personal care homes.

Check the duration of coverage; the elimination periods; and the coverage for adult day care, hospice care, and ambulance service. Be aware that premiums from different companies vary greatly for very similar benefits.

Ask if it is a tax-qualified policy. If so, the premiums one pays may be a tax-deductible medical expense. Look carefully at companies that sell such policies, and choose one whose ratings indicate that it will be there when it is needed. Check the public library for rating publications. Or write for the Special Ratings issue to Insurance Forum, Inc., P.O. Box 245, Ellettsville, Indiana 47429.

Finally, don't procrastinate. One will get a better deal if this insurance is purchased in one's late fifties or early sixties, when one is still in reasonably good health.

If the patient is not prepared to do all this research, consider getting help from a professional to assess the various companies. And I repeat—don't ask your own insurance agent if you expect unbiased advice.

Other Sources of Money

Even if the patient carries insurance, it may be necessary to find other sources of money to pay for his care. In this section, I will discuss a few of the possibilities.

Reverse Mortgages

It may be possible to take out a reverse mortgage on your own or on the patient's home. A reverse mortgage is a loan against one's home that requires no repayment for as long as one lives there. With most loans, the lender checks your income to see how much you can afford to pay back each month. But with a reverse mortgage, you don't have to make monthly repayments, so your income generally has nothing to do with getting the loan.

To get a reverse mortgage,

- You must own your home.
- Everyone who lives in the home must be at least sixty-two years old.

- The home must be your principal residence, which means that you must live in it more than half the year.

The official term for a reverse mortgage is Home Equity Conversion Mortgage (HECM). To qualify for a federally insured HECM, the home must be a single-family property, a two- to four-unit building, or a federally approved condominium or planned unit development. To qualify for Fannie Mae's Home Keeper mortgage, it must be a single-family home or condominium.

Reverse mortgage programs generally do not lend on cooperative apartments or mobile homes. Some manufactured homes may qualify if they are built on a permanent foundation. They must also be classed and taxed as real estate.

If there is any current debt against the home, you must pay it off before getting the reverse mortgage or use a cash advance from the reverse mortgage to clear it. If you don't pay off the debt, or don't qualify for a cash advance large enough to do so, you won't get the mortgage.

There are a number of other ways to produce more money to pay for a health crisis. Ideally, you might prefer not to do some of these things, but if you need the money badly enough, they are worth considering.

Life Insurance Policies

This might be the time for the patient to cash in his life insurance. Most policies allow one to do this, but at a considerable loss. The policyholder can also sell his life insurance by means of a viatical settlement. Under this scheme, a company buys the policyholder's life insurance if he has been diagnosed with a terminal illness. The company will pay about 50 percent of the policy's face value in cash, and it will continue to make the payments on the policy until the policyholder's death.

You need to shop around for the best rates. Call the National Viatical Association in Washington, D.C., to get a list of viatical settlement companies. Their number is (202) 347-7361.

IRAs

If you need extra cash that you can later replace, you can withdraw cash from your IRA account without incurring a penalty as long as you replace it within sixty days. This is called a rollover. You cannot withdraw cash again for twelve months, and you do lose some interest, but an IRA can provide cash in hand when you really need it.

Funds and Foundations

It may also be possible to get some funding, treatment, and equipment free of charge, often through disease foundations or charitable funds such as the following:

- The National Parkinson Foundation (1-800-327-4545) has designated thirteen U.S. Centers of Excellence to treat indigent Parkinson's patients free of charge.
- The ALS Association (1-800-782-4747) will either find or donate medical equipment.
- The American Cancer Society (1-800-227-2345) will both help with finances and lend or donate medical equipment.
- The Leukemia Society (1-800-955-4572) will give financial aid.
- The American Kidney Fund (1-800-638-8299) gives financial aid, while the National Kidney Foundation (1-800-622-9010) gives financial aid and donates or lends medical equipment.
- The American Lung Association (1-800-586-4872) will lend or donate equipment.

A social worker in your local hospital will know which local charities and institutions have equipment to lend or give away.

CHAPTER 5

Legal Responsibilities

One of the most complex issues that caregivers face is that of legal responsibility for a frail or ill elderly person. Generally, once a person cannot manage his own affairs anymore, a spouse or family member assumes day-to-day responsibility for paying bills, taking care of household maintenance, and making arrangements for medical care. Often this person takes over managing all the finances. However, that does not mean that this person has any right to do these things, in a legal sense.

Legal responsibility is seldom planned for, often because the responsible family member feels awkward about raising the subject with her parent or spouse. So in too many families, the subject of legal responsibility is avoided until the last minute, or it never gets dealt with at all. This is not good for anyone.

I cannot stress this enough. Without advance planning, the cost of care for a frail old person can become catastrophic. As I've stated several times in this book, even families that are modestly well off can be wiped out financially trying to pay for medical or nursing home care.

This is not the only reason to plan ahead. Without advance planning, the patient's wishes regarding the type of medical care he wants may be ignored. For example, he could be kept alive on machines against his own and the family's wishes. Patients must clearly express their wishes—in writing—ahead of time.

Without documents legally defining responsibility, the best-intentioned family members may find themselves unable to handle their relative's financial affairs. They may find themselves unable to make decisions about his care without going through the highly distressing process of court hearings. When this happens, the court will appoint an attorney to represent the relative. This leaves the family member in the uncomfortable position of contesting competence and trying to prove that the relative cannot manage his own affairs. The court may even appoint a neutral guardian or conservator rather than a family member to look after the relative's affairs. This guardian or conservator may not agree with family choices for care and could override them.

Finally, it is common for families to take over the finances of an incapacitated parent, even though that parent did not make her wishes known in advance. In families where there are a number of siblings, this can lead to trouble if one sibling accuses another of fraud and embezzlement. Sometimes, again, the issue winds up in court. A well-meaning child may find himself without any legal footing when he thinks he is acting in a responsible way.

In general, only the individual in question has the right to make legal or medical decisions, no matter what his level of competence—unless this responsibility has been legally delegated to someone else. If your elderly relative has not already done so, you need to take the initiative in helping him to make legal plans for the future. Do this no matter how little money he has. Only those with an income below poverty level and no tangible property need not make legal plans for their finances. And everyone needs to make his medical wishes clear.

Sometimes the elderly person is reluctant to do this. She may be reluctant to give up control. She may suspect the motives of anyone who wants to take over for her. It is very important to assure her that no one is trying to take anything away. Perhaps the family member whom she trusts the most, or a lawyer whom she will listen to, can best explain that staying financially safe needs forward planning. And that if she wants her wishes concerning medical treatment to be followed, she must have the appropriate legal documents made out now.

Legal Documents

The minimum legal documents that every person should have in preparation for old age, illness, or incapacity are advance medical directives (also called a living will), medical power of attorney, a will, and financial power of attorney. If the person owns any property, or has any income other than Social Security, he also needs a trust or other legal plan to protect the estate.

Advance Medical Directives

Advance medical directives are documents in which the person defines the type of medical treatment that he wants and states under what circumstances it is to be used. For example, he may foresee the day when he may have Alzheimer's disease and then develop cancer. Under such circumstances, he may not wish to have the cancer treated aggressively.

One of the most important parts of advance medical directives is the section in which the person states whether or not heroic measures are to be used to extend his life. Some people state that they wish to be allowed to die a natural death, rather than to be kept alive by means of resuscitation and machines. Without any clear advance directive on this point, medical intervention must be carried out under the law, even if the family knows that the patient does not want it.

Medical Power of Attorney

The medical power of attorney states the exact circumstances under which a person is given the legal right to make medical decisions for another person. Often the medical power of attorney is included in the advance directives document.

Wills

A person does not need to own much personal property to need a will. The purpose of the will is to state how the person's property—her estate—is to be distributed after she dies. The person may also state what type of funeral or memorial service she wants and how her remains are to be disposed of. A will is a crucial document, the complete plan for settling all of a person's affairs after her death.

Financial Power of Attorney

Financial power of attorney states under what circumstances one person is given the legal right to take over another person's finances, manage his accounts, collect his income, pay his bills, spend his assets, contract debts on his behalf, and so forth. Depending upon the amount of money involved, this right may entail considerable power.

It is crucial to select the right person to exercise this power. Some people choose a family member, while others pick a neutral person. A bank trust officer is often used. Even people who have little more than a monthly pension or Social Security check will want to appoint someone to sign contracts with a care facility, make bank deposits, or pay household bills. Be sure to choose a person whose viewpoints on health and medical choices are similar to your own and who would speak up for you when you can't.

Trusts

A trust is a legal document that is set up to protect a person's assets. It can protect those assets even from an unreliable spouse At all costs, a family must not lose its investments or the property that the person intended to leave them.

Setting Up the Plan

To create any of these documents—and especially to set up a trust—you should consult an attorney who specializes in estate planning. Choose an attorney who is also familiar with federal and state Medicare and Medicaid requirements. There is simply no other way to protect your elderly relative and your family. Only an attorney can sort out the complexities of government regulations. If a private-practice attorney is too expensive, there are free and low-cost legal resources available. These include elder law and estate planning attorneys who offer services through their state bar associations, or through the American Association of Retired Persons.

Legal documents are created for your protection, so they should be easy to locate and readily available to anyone who may need them. Make several copies, and leave the originals with the attorney.

In a serious medical emergency, copies of everything except the will and trust documents must go to the following people:

- All family members, because everyone needs to know what is going on
- All caregivers, so that they know whom to contact, who has authority in case of emergency, and the restrictions listed in the advance medical directives.
- The patient's physician
- The hospital, care facility, or respite program in which the patient resides

Make extra copies of the advance medical directives and both powers of attorney to keep on hand in case of emergency. If, for example, you need to call 911, you will want to have these documents handy. Will and trust documents should be distributed to persons who are trustees and to anyone else that your attorney suggests.

Place copies of important documents under lock and key, so that not just anyone in the house has access to them. These are confidential papers and must be kept secure.

The Patient's Legal Rights

Sometimes ideas about normal, everyday rights collide with what caregivers think is sensible for the person they are looking after. Just as we have the right to decide how we want to live when we are healthy, so too does the patient, even when he is old and sick. Every caregiver should be aware of the legal rights of the elderly, and of her own legal responsibilities as well.

This can be difficult. In our society we often treat old or incapacitated people like children, as if they didn't have the same rights as everyone else. If we are honest with ourselves, we must all admit that we have sometimes done this. How often have we disregarded the dignity of a person who has lost his ability to think clearly? It is easy for us to dominate a helpless or incompetent person—so we must make certain that we don't. As caregivers we must remember that every patient still has all the rights of any citizen, even if we feel that he is no longer acting responsibly or making the choices we expect.

These basic rights are to live where you want to live, to spend your money on what pleases you, to choose your own medical care, and in general to live life in whatever style you choose and can afford. Within the confines of the law, anyone has the right to do anything he pleases, unless he becomes a clear danger to himself or others. This includes the right to refuse to take medicines. Only at the point where the patient's behavior poses a danger are the rest of us legally obligated to interfere for everyone's benefit.

This means that you cannot make your parent do something that she doesn't wish to do. You can't force her into care if she doesn't want to go. And you can't spend her money if she refuses to give it to you. All this is obvious, but generally speaking, this is not where the real problems lie.

The biggest problem area regarding patient's rights is not what happens in families, but what happens in long-term care situations, where the pressures on everyone can seem unbearable. Unfortunately, it is common for caregivers and care staff to violate the rights of residents and patients with the best of intentions—for their own good, so to speak. Sometimes the patient's rights are violated simply because it is convenient for staff. For example, in the past, resident patients were restrained by the use of drugs or actual physical restraints to "keep them safe." All too often, the purpose was actually to keep the patient from walking freely around the place.

As a result of these transgressions, much legislation has been passed in recent years to ensure that everyone respects the rights of residents under long-term care. The Omnibus Budget Reconciliation Act (OBRA) is a federal law that specifies the conditions under which long-term care facilities can receive federal money, such as Medicare and Medicaid funds. OBRA also specifies the rights of patients who reside in these facilities. The OBRA regulations apply in all states, although some states may also have additional regulations.

Long-term care facilities are required to provide the following services to maintain the highest level of well-being for each resident: nursing-related services, rehabilitation services, social services, pharmaceutical services, dietary services, dental services, and treatment of the mentally ill.

In general, each resident of a nursing facility has the right to a dignified existence. Each resident has the right to self-determination. Each resident has the right to communicate with persons and services inside and outside the facility. Residents who are citizens of the United States enjoy all the rights of citizens, and the nursing facility has a duty to protect those rights.

OBRA specifies that

- The resident has the right to be free of interference, coercion, discrimination, and reprisal from the facility in exercising the general rights listed above.
- In the case of a resident who has been adjudged incompetent by a court, the rights of the resident shall be exercised by a person appointed to act on the resident's behalf.
- Any legal surrogate designated in accordance with state law may exercise the resident's rights to the extent provided by state law.
- The facility must inform the resident both orally and in writing, in a language that the resident understands, of his rights and all rules and regulations concerning resident conduct and responsibilities during his stay in the facility. This notice must be made prior to or upon admission to the facility, as well as periodically during the person's stay. The resident must acknowledge in writing that he has received this information.
- The resident has the right to gain access within twenty-four hours (excluding weekends and holidays) to all records pertaining to herself, including current clinical records. The resident has a right to a copy of the records or any portion of the records.
- The resident has the right to be fully informed, in language that he can understand, of his total health status.

- The resident has the right to refuse treatment, to refuse to participate in experimental research, and to formulate advance directives.
- The facility must furnish the resident with a written description of her legal rights.
- The resident has the right not to be abused physically or verbally. Verbal abuse is defined as speaking to a resident in such a way as to detract from the resident's dignity.
- The resident has the right to be neither physically restrained nor restrained by chemicals. Behavior-modifying drugs may be used only with a physician's order, and then only after all other options have been tried and have failed. The fact that other options have failed must be documented.
- The facility must prominently display a notice that describes how to contact the state office of the Long-Term Care Ombudsman. This notice must include the telephone number and usually the Ombudsman's local representative.
- The facility must inform each resident of the name, specialty, and way of contacting the physician who is responsible for his care.
- The facility must provide applicants for admission with oral and written information describing how to apply for and use Medicare and Medicaid benefits and how to receive refunds for previous payments covered by such benefits. This information must be prominently displayed in the facility.
- The facility must immediately inform the resident, consult with the resident's physician, and notify the resident's legal representative or an interested family member, if these persons are known, when the resident is involved in an accident that results in injury and has the potential for requiring physician intervention. The facility must inform when the resident's physical, mental, or psychosocial status deteriorates to a degree that causes a life-threatening

condition or clinical complications; when it becomes necessary to change the resident's treatment significantly; or when a decision has been reached to transfer or discharge the resident from the facility.

- The resident has the right to manage her own financial affairs, and the facility may not require residents to deposit their personal funds with the facility. If a resident does deposit funds with the facility, regulations specify how those funds will be treated and protected.

- Finally, the facility must inform each Medicaid and Medicare resident, in writing, of the items and services that the facility offers for which the resident may not be charged, the items and services that the facility offers for which the resident may be charged, and the costs of the latter. The resident must be informed when any changes are made regarding these items, services, and costs.

During the course of a nursing home stay that is covered by Medicare or Medicaid, the facility may not charge the resident for the following categories of items and services:

- Nursing services
- Dietary services
- Activities programs
- Room and bed maintenance
- Medically related social services
- Items related to personal hygiene (including grooming supplies, incontinence supplies, sanitary napkins, towels and washcloths, hospital gowns, over-the-counter drugs, and personal laundry)

The facility may charge the residents for the following categories of items and services if the resident requests them. The facility must inform the resident that there will be a charge if payment is not made by Medicaid or Medicare:

- Telephone, television, radio for the resident's personal use
- Personal comfort items (including smoking materials, notions, novelties, and confections)
- Cosmetic items
- Clothing
- Reading materials
- Gifts purchased on behalf of the resident
- Flowers and plants
- Social events and entertainment that are not part of the activities program
- Special care services (such as privately hired nurses or aides).
- Private room (except when therapeutically required)
- Specially prepared or alternative food

The facility may not charge a resident (or his representative) for any item or service that the resident has not requested.

Elder Abuse

Family caregivers have an enormous responsibility, and they often feel overburdened. Sometimes this can lead them to neglect, or even abuse, the person they are caring for. This cannot be allowed to continue. If you suspect that an old person is being abused, follow one simple rule: Call for help.

The following are signs of possible abuse:

- Malnourished or dishevelled physical appearance (being dirty, missing glasses or dentures, wearing torn or ragged clothing)
- Physical injuries (bruises, burns, welts, rope burns, bed sores, tufts of hair missing, broken bones) for which there is

no adequate explanation. Also be suspicious of multiple injuries in different stages of healing.

- Withdrawn, apathetic, fearful behavior. Notice especially if the old person seems fearful around certain people.
- A sudden change in the old person's standard of living, especially if his financial assets are being depleted without explanation. He may be the victim of elder fraud. Someone with diminished judgment can fall prey to unscrupulous people who steal his money. It is also the caregiver's responsibility to look out for this kind of abuse.

If you find that the person is in imminent danger, she should be removed from the situation immediately. The police should be notified. Contact doctors, psychologists, lawyers, social workers, bank officials, and so forth and ask them to assist in the investigation. (Note that most states require health care professionals to report suspected elder abuse to the legal authorities.)

If you suspect that a nursing home resident is being abused by the staff, file an official complaint with the staff supervisor, the director of the home, and the resident's doctor. Contact the local Agency on Aging for additional information and assistance. Most importantly, call the local or state office of the Long-Term Care Ombudsman. For further information, contact:

National Center on Elder Abuse (NCEA)
c/o American Public Welfare Association
810 First Street, N.E.
Washington, D.C. 20002
(202) 682-2470
www.gwjapan.com/NCEA

American Association of Retired Persons
601 East Street, N.W.
Washington, D.C. 20049
(202) 434-2277; 1-800-424-3410
www.aarp.org

A Caregiver's Responsibilities

With respect to the patient's rights, the legal responsibilities of the in-home professional caregiver are very much the same as those of the institutional caregiver. Because as in-home caregiver you are often alone with a person who may be forgetful or incompetent, it is crucial that you be scrupulous in avoiding anything that could be even vaguely construed as abusive. You must also take scrupulous precautions regarding the procedures you use to protect and account for the patient's valuables and money. Keep a written record of every transaction.

Before we leave the subject of legal responsibilities, let's look briefly at the caregiver's responsibilities to herself. Caregivers are often expected to do an extreme amount of work for very little pay. This will continue until professional caregivers are willing to demand better compensation. I suggest that you do the following things.

Ask for at least minimum hourly wage in addition to room and board. The law requires employers to file withholding tax and pay health insurance on employees. Because most caregivers prefer to act as independent contractors, taxes on their wages are not withheld, and they must pay for their own health insurance. If you agree to be paid by twenty-four-hour shift, typical charges currently range from $100 to $130 per day.

Carefully define the work expected of you. Do not agree to do housework without defining whether this means routine tidying or heavy cleaning. Do not agree to do all the shopping and cooking if you are also charged with supervising a patient who might wander off if left unattended. Do not agree to provide services such as minor nursing unless you are legally qualified to do so. It is a good idea to have a written contract that defines your job responsibilities.

Carefully define the exact hours you are expected to work and the time you have off. This is especially important if you are a live-in caregiver. It is too easy to slip into providing help just because no one else is around, or to be expected to provide help on your day off just because you happen to be in the home.

Protect yourself from burnout. Remember that you are an employee with your own legal rights. Unfortunately, your employer may not respect those rights unless you insist. (You have the right to sue for these rights, but this is unlikely to happen.)

CHAPTER 6

Death Comes as the End

After we are born, the only other guaranteed major event in our lives is that we will die. How surprising that we sometimes still pretend that this will not happen! Doctors talk about extending human life, as if this would somehow remove the possibility of death. Many people avoid being with a dying person. Even the language of death has become evasive—instead of dying, people pass on, pass away, transcend. Some people even manage never to go to a funeral. In this chapter, I am going to talk about dealing with death.

Once they know that their illness is terminal, many people want to decide where they will die. These days, one can die in a hospital, in long-term care, or at home. Even in a hospital, one can decide to come home at any time. It is often best to plan ahead. If you are caring for a terminal patient, the decision as to where he will die may actually be yours.

Most of us feel apprehensive about the death of someone we care about. If you really don't think you can manage caregiving for someone at home, don't make yourself do it. But don't be too quick to assume that you can't. Remember that you can get a great deal of help from hospice. The hospice home nurses will be able to teach you things that you need to know, and they will help you on a daily basis. You will not be left alone to provide the patient with difficult nursing care. You will have someone on call night and day for emergencies or advice.

In America, the subject of death—when it is talked about at all—is becoming romanticized. The notion is that everyone will have a fully conscious, self-realized attitude about facing death. This is far from reality. In fact, people tend to die the way they have lived. People who are emotionally honest and courageous face death most easily. People who have been afraid to live are usually also afraid to die. This can sometimes make it difficult to talk about choices.

Many dying people do not want to admit that they are dying. They avoid conversation, refuse to hear hints, and are set on seeing a doctor and getting better. This makes sense, given that survival is a primal urge. But on the other hand, people who are in denial are likely to struggle a lot in the dying process. Even when they are medicated, they are restless and disturbed. They constantly try to get out of bed and get away. They may kick, struggle, and cry out for help to escape.

This can be disturbing for the caregiver, especially if she is not sure what to do. As a caregiver, your main task will be to center yourself and know that you are doing all that can be done. If the patient is sufficiently medicated and not in physical pain, the death process will take care of itself.

There are usually long, slow periods when the patient seems to be meditating or dreaming. Often she will utter an odd sentence that means nothing, except to her. Maybe she has something on her mind. Be alert to listen for signals.

"I've failed at everything I've ever done in my life." I once heard these words from an old man as he lay dying. Outwardly, he seemed successful enough. A long and happy marriage, a prosperous job, no major glitches in life, apparently—but this was not his emotional truth. He had actually concealed many things from others—and perhaps from himself—until he lay dying.

I knew that I had to let him share this hard realization. While taking him for a drive by the river, I began to tell him about all the ways he had succeeded in other people's eyes—his generosity, the way he had inspired his students, and his kindness. I hope that he learned to value himself before he died.

The Predeath Vigil

As death becomes imminent, home care really requires that two people be available most of the time, even though there are likely to be long, quiet times, as I have just explained. Should the patient need physical help, it will be easier with two of you there.

Make plans beforehand to obtain everything you will need. Ask hospice nurses to help you to make a list. For example, get a hospital bed, a commode chair, a wheelchair, rubber rings for the patient to sit on, or maybe lambskins or an egg crate mattress for extra comfort. Most of these things will be available on Medicare or Medicaid. The patient's doctor will write a prescription, or you can hire the equipment and submit the receipts to the patient's insurance company. Some of these items are so cheap that you could buy them from a department store like Wal-Mart. Wheelchairs can be found free locally, or a friend may have one. (Once when we needed a wheelchair, we were offered three from people's garages or storerooms.)

Talk to the patient's doctor about the probable course of the final stages of the illness. Review the patient's advance medical directives with the doctor. Raise the question of pain medication, and get the doctor's assurance that the patient will not be allowed to be in pain.

Death Away from Home

While it is possible that the patient may die in the hospital, it is also possible that he may die in a nursing home, or even in a hospice. If the patient is fortunate enough to die in a hospice, he will get full attention, respect, and help with the dying process.

If he dies in a nursing home, this is less likely. Many nursing homes have absolutely no special programs for residents who are dying, and so these residents often die alone. The staff may simply leave them to die, not turning them every two hours as they are supposed to, or making sure that their pain medication is appropriate. Staff members have even been known to decide arbitrarily to cut down on this medication. On the East Coast, a nursing home and a doctor were recently sued successfully for leaving a ninety-two-year-old terminal cancer patient in constant pain, despite the pleas of her relatives. The doctor's excuse was "Well, you don't want your mother to become addicted to morphine, do you?" The fact that the woman was dying in agony had no effect. The woman died; the family brought suit and won; and the doctor was suspended from practice. A substantial monetary judgment was leveled against the nursing home.

Before choosing a nursing home, therefore, be sure to ask the officials the following questions about their policy for dying patients:

- When was the last time you had a workshop on death and dying for your staff?
- What is your policy on increasing pain medication when the patient continues to be in pain?
- What is your care routine for the dying?
- What is your ratio of staff to patients on each shift?
- How do you ensure privacy for the dying patient and his family?

If you have any doubts, you might think about calling in hospice to help care for the patient in the nursing home. Medicare and Medicaid both give you this right. Pick a nursing home that seems receptive to this, with a nursing director who seems to be aware that dying patients have special needs.

Do as many things as you can to make the patient's room warm and special. Bring treasured photographs, bedcovers from home, books, perhaps music CDs. The patient will be comfortable around familiar things. Find out if you can have a rollaway bed, so you can stay in the room with the patient when death is imminent. This will help the patient feel emotionally comfortable.

The Dying Process

The actual dying process can seem interminable. Yet during this time, old family business can be taken care of. In families whose members are estranged, this can be a time of reconciliation. An angry, distant son may refuse to come to his father's deathbed; a sister may still not want to forgive her brother after forty years. In such cases, the caregiver can sometimes act as a peacemaker.

Consider how to make sure that the patient has the power of choice in all things, including the atmosphere of his final environment. Does he want music in his room, or silence? Something that smells good? Favorite foods? A special book read to him? A cat on the bed? Organize bringing in any of these requests.

Remember that a peaceful human presence is deeply comforting to the dying person. Some patients might want to hold your hand. Others may want to be left alone, but they will all probably appreciate your just being there.

A dying person gradually eats and drinks less. You should not be alarmed when this happens. Offer easy-to-digest nourishment—yogurts, custards, or light soups. Water is the best liquid, but give the patient whatever she can keep down. Family members should not panic and feel that the patient should eat more at all costs. Her body's systems are closing down. You can help by providing simple comforts. Gently dab dry lips with a moist cotton swab. Ice chips to suck can also be very comforting.

From the time the patient stops eating entirely, it could take him up to three weeks to die. Even after he stops drinking, he may survive as many as ten days—a surprisingly long time. During this stage, the body's struggle to close down can seem like a battle to stay alive. It is distressing to watch. The patient may be fighting to breathe, may pluck restlessly at the sheets, or may even try to get out of bed, although he is too weak. Maybe some extra oxygen would help, or morphine to ease the pain.

Doctors often forget to reduce the ordinary medication of a dying person—for example, by withdrawing diuretics in a person who is not even drinking. Hospice nurses are skilled in advising doctors unfamiliar with the intimate processes of death. But generally, you will have to raise all these questions yourself. Try to find out what you can about the dying process.

As death draws near, the patient will lose heat from the extremities, especially from the feet and legs. He may enter what is known as Cheyne-Stokes breathing—long, deep breaths separated by gaps, followed by shallow, panting breaths. This can come and go in the days before death. The patient may seem flushed and feverish at one time, yellowish and chilled at another. These are all the signs that death is imminent.

You may have heard of the death rattle, the sound that a person makes when he is close to death. This harsh, guttural, throat-wrenching sound is made by the accumulation of mucus in the throat. It may continue for hours, or even whole days. It is a very distinctive sound, yet not a sound of pain. It is important to remember that most of the dying struggle you may witness is probably not felt as distress or pain.

As death approaches, you will often hear the patient talking to someone who isn't there. This is a normal phenomenon, and caregivers with faith find it very comforting because it seems to confirm their belief in an afterlife. Listen with acceptance if the patient discusses it.

Death can come very suddenly. However, in the case of a protracted illness, it is usually so gradual that families and caregivers have time to get used to the idea. If you are feeling nervous about the effect that death will have on the patient's appearance, you could do some reading on death and dying to come to terms with it and to know what to expect. If you have spiritual beliefs, this will help the caregiver to come to terms with the effect of death on the patient's appearance and by making the process of dying familiar instead of strange and frightening.

Many people stay with the dying person day and night; then, just in the five minutes when they slip next door to get a cup of coffee, the person actually dies. This is ironic, but it is very common. An oncology nurse once told me, "I think it's hard for the dying person to leave their family. So it's in the time someone is away that this person is free to go. Often it's when the family has gone home for the night. The patient has picked his time."

Finally, remember that, even if the patient seems to be in a coma, recent research indicates that she is in fact deeply conscious. This means that you can talk to her and share things. Tell her that you love her. Try not to be timid or afraid.

At the first death I experienced, a ninety-seven-year-old woman was semicomatose after a major stroke. Aware that somehow their mother was still clinging to life, her two daughters knelt one on each side of her bed. One of them said, "Mom, you remember how you used to take us sledding when we were kids? Remember how you'd take us to the top of the hill?"

The second daughter joined in, "That's right, Mom. I'd always be so scared, and you'd say it was okay, that I should just let go and slide down; it'll be easy. Well, Mom, this is like that now. You've climbed and climbed, yourself. Now you can just let go and slide down. There's nothing to be scared of. Just let go . . ."

Within twenty minutes, after hanging on for ten days, their mother finally died. A loving end to a long struggle.

One Last Checklist

You should do some of these things as soon as you realize that the patient is dying. You should do the others immediately after he has died.

- Let the mortuary know that the patient is expected to die shortly.
- Contact the patient's doctor. The doctor must see the patient no more than two months before his death. Otherwise, the law requires that an autopsy be performed. If the doctor has seen the patient and agrees that death is imminent, there will be no problem about getting a death certificate.
- If you want the body moved immediately, call the mortuary; they will usually show up within half an hour. On the other hand, if you want to keep the person at home for one last night, you may do so.
- Send copies of the death certificate to Social Security, to the patient's insurance company, and to anyone else who needs official confirmation of the patient's death.

- If your name is on the patient's bank account and you want to withdraw money, you must do so before you notify the bank of the death. After the bank has been officially notified, the account will be frozen.

Grieving

In the first few days following the death, you will have a lot to do. You may have to telephone or write to many people, and you will probably play host to others as well. It may be a few days before the full extent of your loss hits you emotionally. You may want company then; many people choose to be with family and friends. Or you may find it more peaceful to be alone.

If you dearly loved the person who has died, of course you will grieve—and you will do it in whatever way comes naturally to you. Don't let anyone tell you how you "ought" to feel, although it is good to have someone to confide in. (Sometimes insensitive people will even tell you to "get over it." Just ignore them.)

Often, people report that after some weeks or even months, they are suddenly hit by a great tidal wave of grief. You are very likely to find birthdays, anniversaries, or holidays painful. It is normal to feel sad at the approach of the date when your person passed away. During these times, do whatever feels appropriate. Weep, or spend time alone, or seek the comfort of others—whatever brings you peace.

You should not make rash decisions on important matters after the death of someone you love. Do not sell your house; don't move away; don't remarry too quickly. Give yourself time to feel. Wait to make important decisions until your emotions are again in balance.

Be aware that when you have been looking after someone intensely for so long, you may feel that you could have done things better. You may feel guilty, remembering moments when you were impatient or irritable. Sometimes you may have lost control of your emotions because you were tired, frustrated, or scared. It is important to be kind to yourself about these things. Don't add to your pain by blaming yourself. No one is perfect. You did the best you could, and that is as much as anyone can do.

If you walked with someone through a horrible illness to the gates of death, that was an admirable commitment and sacrifice on your part. You deserve praise for having done such a wonderful thing.

Finding In-Home Services

The following agencies and organizations offer many different kinds of support services. These services can make the difference between being able to keep a person at home and having to choose out-of-home placement.

IN-HOME SERVICES AND GENERAL INFORMATION

AARP Fulfillment
601 East Street, N.W.
Washington, D.C. 20049
1-800-424-3410
(Twenty-page booklet: Care Management: Arranging for Long-Term Care.
   Order #D13803. Provides information on selecting and evaluating
   geriatric care management services.)

Adventures in Movement for the Handicapped (AIM)
945 Danbury Road
Dayton, Ohio 45420
(513) 294-4611
(For the disabled and their family caregivers, AIM is a specialized
   movement education program taught to music.)

American Association of Homes and Services for the Aging
(AAHSA)
901 East Street, N.W.
Suite 500
Washington, D.C. 20004
(202) 783-2242
(National association for over five thousand not-for-profit nursing homes,
   health-related facilities, and community service organizations for the
   elderly. Helpful free publications. Send a self-addressed stamped envelope
   for each copy: Assisted Living, Offering Supportive Care for the Older
   Adult, Choosing a Nursing Home, A Guide to Quality Care, The
   Continuous CareRetirement Community.)

American Association of Retired Persons (AARP)
601 East Street, N.W.
Washington, D.C. 20049
(202) 434-2120
(Telephone hot lines offering free legal consultation for callers aged sixty
   and over.)

American Bar Association
Commission on Legal Problems of the Elderly
(202) 662-8690
Concern for the Dying
(212) 366-5440
(Provides information on living wills.)

American Institute of Certified Public Accountants
1211 Avenue of the Americas
New York, New York 10036
1-800-862-4270
(Provides information on estate and financial planning, plus local referrals.)

American Safe Deposit Association
330 West Main Street
Greenwood, Indiana 46142
(317) 888-1118
(Provides help in determining whether a deceased person had a safe-deposit box.)

Assistance Pension Rights Center
918 Sixteenth Street, N.W.
Suite 704
Washington, D.C. 20006
(202) 296-3776
(Provides information and guidance.)

Assisted Living Facilities Association of America
(703) 691-8100
(Provides information and publications.)

Children of Aging Parents
1-800-227-7294

Concerned Relatives of Nursing Home Patients
(216) 321-0403
(Provides information regarding nursing home placement, Medicare, and Medicaid.)

Disabled Hotline: Direct Link
(805) 688-1603
(Provides information from 12,000 local organizations.)

Eldercare Locator
c/o Administration of Aging
United States Department of Health and Human Services
1-800-677-1116, Monday through Friday, 9:00 A.M. to 8:00 P.M. EST.
(A nationwide directory assistance service operated and funded by the federal government. Designed to help older persons and caregivers locate local support resources for aging Americans. You will get information on how to locate a wide variety of services: meals, home care transportation, housing alternatives, home repair, recreation, social activities, and legal services. Will also provide you with the names and phone numbers of organizations within a desired location, anywhere in the country.)

Elder Helpline
1-800-262-2243
(Provides referrals to local agencies and general information.)

Elderly Homeowner Rehabilitation Program (EHR)
Consult local telephone directory.
(Provides grants for making deferred loans for home rehabilitation. State Health and Rehabilitative Services may also provide these grants.)

Fraud Hot Line (HHSA Tips)
P.O. Box 23489
Washington, D.C. 20026
1-800-447-8477
(Hot line for reporting crime committed by health service workers or programs.)

Generations United
c/o Child Welfare League of America
440 First Street, N.W.
Suite 310
Washington, D.C. 20001-2085
(202) 638-4004
(National coalition of more than 130 organizations and volunteers who help frail, homebound, older people to live more independently.)

Health Care Financing Administration
U.S. Department of Health and Human Services
200 Independence Avenue, S.W.
Washington, D.C. 20201
1-800-772-1213
(Provides information and free publications: Guide to Health Insurance for People with Medicare, Medicare and Advance Directives, Medicare Handbooks.)

Health Insurance Association of America
1-800-635-1271
(Provides information, a list of companies that offer long-term care insurance, and a free publication: Guide to Long-Term Care Insurance.)

Legal Counsel for the Elderly
American Association of Retired Persons (AARP)
1-800-424-3410
(Provides hot lines, free legal advice, and local referrals to low-cost legal help.)

Living Bank
1-800-528-2971
(Provides information on organ donation.)

Medicare Hot Line
1-800-638-6833
(Provides free information, answers questions, reports Medicare fraud.)

Menu Direct Corporation 865
1-888-MENU123
(Menu Direct is a corporation that can provide diabetic meals, and other special diet foods delivered to your door, ready to heat and eat. Consulting nutritionists on the phone.)

National Academy of Elder Law Attorneys
(602) 881-4005

National Adult Day Services Association
c/o National Council on Aging (NCOA)
409 Third Street, S.W.
Suite 200
Washington, D.C. 20024
(202) 479-1200
(Free publications: NCOA Resources Guide, Your Guide to Selecting an Adult Day Center.)

National Association of Meal Programs
(703) 548-5558
(Provides information for providers and local referrals for community dining and in-home meal services. A membership organization.)

National Association of Professional Geriatric Care Managers (GCM)
750 First Street, N.E.
Tucson, Arizona 85716
(502) 881-8008

National Citizen's Coalition of Nursing Home Reform
(202) 332-2275
(Provides information, advocacy, guidance in selecting a nursing home, and local referrals.)

National Clearinghouse for Legal Services, Inc.
205 Monroe Street, Second Floor
Chicago, Illinois 60606
(312) 263-3830
(Provides publications on health, senior citizens, and housing.)

National Council on Aging (NCOA)
409 Third Street, S.W.
Suite 200
Washington, D.C. 20024
1-800-424-9046; 1-800-292-3513
(Provides help regarding issues related to aging services and adult day care.)

National Family Caregivers Association
9621 E. Bexhill Drive
Kensington, Maryland 20895-3104
1-800-896-3650

National Insurance Consumers Helpline
1-800-942-4242
(Provides information and referrals regarding Medicare; long-term care; and health, home, auto, and business insurance.)

National Meals on Wheels Foundation
1-800-999-6262
(Provides grants to meal programs, meal delivery, volunteer referrals, and a service hot line.)

National Self-Help Clearinghouse
City University of New York
25 W. Forty-Third Street
Room 620
New York, New York 10036

Nursing Home Information Service
National Council of Senior Citizens
1331 F Street, N.W.
Washington, D.C. 20004
(202) 347-8800, Ext. 340

Rosalynn Carter Institute
Georgia Southwestern College
800 Wheatley Street
Americus, Georgia 31709-4693
(912) 928-1234

Senior Net
1 Kearny Street, Third Floor
San Francisco, California 94108
(415) 352-1210

Social Security Administration
1-800-772-1213
(Free publications: Understanding Social Security, SSI Supplemental Security Income. Provides legal assistance with wills, trusts, powers of attorney, living wills; provides financial and insurance resources.)

United Seniors Health Cooperative
(202) 662-8690
(Nonprofit organization, provides information regarding insurance, referrals, publications, and more to help the elderly lead healthy, independent lives.)

Veteran's Administration (VA)
1-800-827-1000
(Provides benefits of all kinds for qualified veterans.)

HEALTH AND EDUCATION

Alzheimer's Association
Centennial Avenue
Piscataway, New Jersey 08854
1-800-272-3900
*(Provides nationwide referrals to local chapters, services, and support
   groups.)*

Cancer Care Counseling Line
1-800-813-4673, 9:00 A.M. to 5:00 P.M. EST.
E-mail: info@cancercare.org
*(Callers will be connected to an oncology social worker, who will provide
   counseling, referrals, and information. Cancer Care also runs
   educational programs and support groups over the phone. Ask questions
   via E-mail.)*

National AIDS Clearinghouse
1-800-458-5231

National AIDS Hot Line
1-800-342-2437
*(Provides referrals to legal, financial, and medical resources; support
   groups; and publications. Sponsored by Centers for Disease Control.)*

National Alliance of Breast Cancer Organizations
1-800-719-9154
(Provides information, support, and publications.)

National Rehabilitation Information Center
8455 Colesvileel Road
Suite 935
Silver Spring, Maryland 20910
1-800-346-2742
*(Federally funded. Provides database information on equipment and home
   modification and referrals to local rehabilitation centers and
   organizations that provide help for the disabled.)*

National Spinal Cord Injury Association
1-800-526-3456
(Provides referrals to rehabilitation programs, clinics, equipment centers, support groups, and publications.)

Parkinson's Disease Foundation
1-800-457-6676
(Provides educational information and referrals to support groups by zip code, and sponsors research.)

Visiting Nurse Associations of America
1-800-426-2547
(Central listing to locate your nearest Visiting Nurse Association, which will manage and coordinate the details of in-home hospice care.)

Y-Me National Breast Cancer Organization
1-800-221-2141
(Provides information, counseling, referrals to doctors and clinics, and support for patients and partners; provides publications.)

HOSPICE

Choice in Dying
200 Varick Street
New York, New York 10014-0148
1-800-989-WILL
(Provides state-specific living wills and durable powers of attorney.)

Hospice Association of America
519 C Street, N.E.
Washington, D.C. 20002
(202) 546-4759
(Provides publications about hospice services.)

National Hospice Organization
Hospice Hot Line
1-800-658-8898
(Provides comprehensive emotional, spiritual, physical, and social services to terminally ill patients and their families. Offers compassionate care for patients, information, and publications. Also provides local referrals.)

Caregiver Education

As a caregiver, you must learn as much as possible about the disease of the person you're caring for. Information can come from many places, but it is generally true that the best education comes from experience. People who live and work with patients on a daily basis have the most to share.

Although it is important to have technical knowledge about a disease, ultimately you need answers to questions that arise daily in your hands-on work. Fortunately, many support groups, associations, and information groups have been formed to educate the public. Some of the most important ones are listed on the following pages.

ILLNESSES, DISEASES, DISABILITIES

Alzheimer's Association
1-800-272-3900
(Provides nationwide referrals to local chapters, services, and support groups.)

Alzheimer's Disease Education and Referral Center
1-800-438-4390
(Provides free information on Alzheimer's and other dementia-related diseases.)

American Brain Tumor Association
1-800-886-2282
(Provides referrals to doctors, support groups, and publications.)

American Cancer Society
1-800-227-2345
(Provides free information, publications, and referrals; answers personal questions.)

American Cancer Society Hot Line
1-800-ACS-2345
(Provides local referrals.)

American Diabetes Association
1-800-868-7888
(Provides information and local referrals.)

American Heart Association
National Center and Stroke Connection
1-800-242-8721; 1-800-553-6321
(Provides free publications.)

American Lung Association
1-800-586-4872
(Provides information on all aspects of lung diseases and local referrals for medical care, smoking cessation, and support groups.)

American Lupus Foundation
1-800-331-1802
(Provides an information packet.)

American Parkinson's Disease Association
1-800-223-3732
(Provides publications and local referrals.)

Arthritis Foundation
1-800-283-7800
(Provides free information and nationwide referral to local chapters and support groups.)

Asthma and Allergy Foundation of America
1-900-727-8462
(Provides publications and referrals to other hot lines.)

Cancer Care
1-800-813-HOPE

Leukemia Society of America
1-800-955-4572
(Provides referrals to local chapters, publications, and a newsletter.)

Lupus Foundation of America
1-800-558-0121
(Provides information and referrals to local chapters.)

National Alliance of Breast Cancer Organizations
1-800-719-9154
(Provides information, support, and publications.)

National Cancer Institute
9000 Rockville Pike
31 Center Drive
MSC 2580
Bethesda, Maryland 20892-2580
(301) 496-5583; 1-800-422-6237; 1-800-332-8615

National Coalition for Cancer Survivorship
1010 Wayne Avenue
Silver Spring, Maryland 20910
(301) 650-8868

National Institute of Neurological Disorders and Stroke
1-800-352-9424
(Provides nationwide referrals to local centers and information on Alzheimer's, epilepsy, Parkinson's, stroke, and other brain-related disorders.)

National Organization for Rare Disorders
1-800-999-6673
*(Provides information and local referrals. First request is free. A nonprofit
clearinghouse.)*

Parkinson's Disease Foundation
1-800-457-6676
*(Provides educational information and referrals to support groups by zip
code, and sponsors research.)*

Y-Me National Breast Cancer Organization
1-800-221-2141
*(Provides information, counseling, referrals to doctors and clinics, support
for patients and their partners, and publications.)*

CAREGIVER ORGANIZATIONS

These organizations provide caregiver information, and may also
provide support groups, newsletters, conferences, and workshops for
caregivers.

Bone Marrow Transplant Family Support Network
1-800-826-9376

Cancer Care Counseling Line
1-800-813-4673
E-mail: info@cancercare.org
*(Callers are connected to an oncology social worker, who provides counseling,
information, referrals, teleconference information, and other services.
Also runs educational programs and support groups over the phone.)*

Candlelighters Childhood Cancer Foundation
1-800-366-2223

Child Health Resource Line
1-800-400-PEDS

Children of Parkinsonians
(760) 773-5628

Diabetes Educator Access Line
1-800-832-6874

Intercommunity Caregivers
(303) 778-5984

Multiple Sclerosis Information Resource Center
1-800-344-4867

Multiple Sclerosis Foundation
1-800-441-7055

National Academy of Elder Law Attorneys
(520) 881-4005

National Alliance for the Mentally Ill
1-800-950-6264

National Association for Sickle Cell Disease
1-800-421-8453

National Brain Tumor Foundation
1-800-934-2873

National Head Injury Foundation
1-800-444-6443

Spina Bifida Association
1-800-621-3141

Stroke Connection
1-800-553-6321

DEATH AND DYING

American Academy of Hospice and Palliative Medicine
P.O. Box 14288
Gainesville, Florida 32604-2288
(352) 377-8900

Association for Death Education and Counseling
638 Prospect Avenue
Hartford, Connecticut 06105
(203) 232-4825

Family Caregiver Alliance
425 Bush Street
Suite 500
San Francisco, California 94108
(415) 434-3388

Family Caregiver Project
University of North Carolina at Charlotte
Department of Psychology
Charlotte, North Carolina 28223
(704) 547-4758
*(Provides manuals on caregiving, particular illnesses, and a publication:
Caring Families: Dying and Death.)*

Foundation for Hospice and Homecare
320 A Street, N.E.
Washington, D.C. 20002
(202) 547-6586
(Provides information and a free publication: All About Hospice.)

Hospice Nurses Association
Medical Center East
211 N. Whitfield Street
Suite 375
Pittsburgh, Pennsylvania 15206-3031
(412) 361-2474

National Association of Home Care (NAHC)
228 Seventh Street, S.E.
Washington, D.C. 20003-4360
(202) 547-5277

National Hospice Organization
1901 N. Moore Street
Suite 901
Arlington, Virginia 22209
(703) 243-5900

Internet Resources

It is not always easy to locate resources within your own community, and your work as a caregiver may not leave you with much time to look. Fortunately, there is a wealth of data available in your home via the Internet. (Computers are also widely available in your public library.) These resources are truly impressive and are free for the taking.

An effective way to get what you need is to use the appropriate keywords for your search—for example, "Alzheimer's," "HMOs," "care homes." This extends your possible range of information a great deal. If there is too much information for you to make written notes, remember to bookmark the site. This keeps it easily available for future reference. Or simply print out the pages you need.

www.acor.org

Association of Cancer On-Line Resources (ACOR). An umbrella for on-line support groups and information groups for dealing with cancer. A great resource.

www.aidsinfobbs.org

A database of information on all aspects of AIDS. Publications, reports, medical reviews of treatment.

www.alz.org

The site for the Alzheimer's Association. Provides access to the services of the association, plus a list of chapters throughout the United States and a list of support groups with schedules of meetings. Many states also have hot lines that you can call for advice.

www.caregiver.org

The focus of this site is obvious from the name. As a caregiver, you will find a lot of help here.

www.drugstore.com

A useful commercial Web site that can make the caregiver's life a lot easier. It includes a complete pharmacy, with a fine selection of homeopathic medicines, as well as many personal care products, all delivered to your door at very reasonable prices.

    This site also has an up-to-date drug index that lists thousands of prescription medications, tells what they are used for, and lists precautions, interactions, and side effects. There is also an on-line pharmacist to answer your questions.

www.fly.hiwaay.net/^bparris/alzmnews

A personal site by a woman who cared for her mother, an Alzheimer's patient, created in memory of that hard year.

www.Geocities.com/HotSprings/1159

My Alzheimer's help page, an alternative approach to understanding patients with dementia, using natural resources. A forum for people to talk with one another. (Cited as a two-star site by web.md and highlighted as a Geocities special site.)

www.healthguide.com

This site provides a wealth of information in the following categories: brain, body, family, senior, pharmacy, and professional.

www.mayohealth.org
This is the Mayo Clinic's Web site. It provides extensive material on
health and illness and very good basic information for caregivers.

www.medicare.gov
This excellent Web site provides in-depth guides to Medicare,
Medicaid, health insurance, and every licensed nursing home in
the United States.

www.Mentalhelp.net
A guide to mental health issues, including dementia and depression, with
an excellent on-line bookstore and access to free therapy.

www.my.webmd.com
This excellent site provides health guidance on general topics and areas of
interest, such as Alzheimer's, arthritis, cancer, and prescription drugs.
Chat rooms where you can communicate with others, including on-
line experts.

www.nlm.nih.gov
The National Institute of Health's huge site provides access to searchable
sources of medical and health information.
It includes the Visible Human Project. It also includes Grateful
Med (aka Medline). This great resource is an index and summary of
almost every article published in every medical journal in the world.
You can find information by topic, author, or title. A synopsis of each
article is included. Instructions on how to use the site are posted.
Excellent for in-depth research. And it's free.

www.senior.com
This site has everything you could ever need on medical, help, housing,
and legal issues for seniors.

www.seniorlaw.com
A guide to elder law, including estates, Medicare and Medicaid, and the
legal rights of old people.

www.senioroptions.com
Maintained by a nonprofit organization, this site is a guide to resources
in a number of categories: senior living options, legal help, caregiver
resources, and so forth. For each category, there is a list of specific
resources, searchable by city, county, and state.

www.Suite101.com

This magazine-style help site is especially strong in Alzheimer's care. Very informative and easy to use.

www.sympatico.ca/healthyway/feature_alz3.html

General help and guidance for a wide range of diseases and needs, from Alzheimer's to terminal illness caregiving. Well organized and easy to use.

www.thebody.com

This site deals with every aspect of AIDS and HIV. It hosts over forty information, self-help, and support groups and sets up free interactive chats with experts.

www.virtuallawoffice.com

This site is a legal advice service offering support, care, and help for families on legal and financial matters.

www.webmd.com

This is one of the better on-line sources for medical information, including information on alternative health. It has a library of medical books and articles, a question-and-answer site, and chat sites on specific topics. It also includes on-line support programs, such as Smoker's Cessation.

State Agencies on Aging

Forty-two states and Puerto Rico have federal Area Agencies on Aging (AAAs), which are part of the governmental supervisory and referral services for elders in this country. The rest of the states have state agencies.

Every person should know how to contact his local AAA office. Telephone numbers are usually listed in local telephone directories. The following information may also be helpful.

ALABAMA
Region IV
Alabama Commission on Aging
RSA Plaza
Suite 470
770 Washington Avenue
Montgomery, Alabama
  36130-1851
(334) 242-5743
FAX: (334) 242-5594

ALASKA
Region X
Alaska Commission on Aging
Division of Senior Services
Department of Administration
Juneau, Alaska 99811-0209
(907) 465-3250
FAX: (907) 465-4716

ARIZONA
Region IX
Aging and Adult Administration
Department of Economic Security
1789 W. Jefferson Street
Suite 950A
Phoenix, Arizona 85007
(602) 542-4446
FAX: (602) 542-6575

ARKANSAS
Region VI
Division Aging and Adult Services
Arkansas Dept of Human Services
1417 Donaghey Plaza South
P.O. Box 1437, Slot 1412
Little Rock, Arkansas 72203-1437
(501) 682-2441
FAX: (501) 682-8155

CALIFORNIA
Region IX
California Department of Aging
1600 K Street
Sacramento, California 95814
(916) 322-5290
FAX: (916) 324-1903

COLORADO
Region VIII
Aging and Adult Services
Department of Social Services
110 Sixteenth Street
Suite 200
Denver, Colorado 80202-4147
(303) 620-4147
FAX: (303) 620-4191

CONNECTICUT
Region I
Division of Elderly Services
25 Sigourney Street, Tenth Floor
Hartford, Connecticut
  06106-5033
(860) 424-5277
FAX: (860) 424-4966

DELAWARE
Region III
Delaware Division of Services for
  Aging and Adults with Physical
  Disabilities
Department of Health and Social
  Services
1901 North DuPont Highway
New Castle, Delaware 19720
(302) 577-4791
FAX: (302) 577-4793

DISTRICT OF COLUMBIA
Region III
District of Columbia Office on
    Aging
One Judiciary Square,
    Ninth Floor
441 Fourth Street, N.W.
Washington, D.C. 20001
(202) 724-5622
FAX: (202) 724-4979

FLORIDA
Region IV
Department of Elder Affairs
Building B
Suite 152
4040 Esplanade Way
Tallahassee, Florida 32399-7000
(904) 414-2000
FAX: (904) 414-2004

GEORGIA
Region IV
Division of Aging Services
Department of Human Resources
2 Peachtree Street, N.E.,
    Thirty-Sixth Floor
Atlanta, Georgia 30303-3176
(404) 657-5258
FAX: (404) 657-5285

GUAM
Region IX
Division of Senior Citizens
Department of Public Health &
    Social Services
P.O. Box 2816
Agana, Guam 96910
(671) 475-0263
FAX: (671) 477-2930

HAWAII
Region IX
Hawaii Executive Office on Aging
250 S. Hotel Street
Suite 109
Honolulu, Hawaii 96813-2831
(808) 586-0100
FAX: (808) 586-0185

IDAHO
Region X
Idaho Commission on Aging
P.O. Box 83720
Boise, Idaho 83706
(208) 334-3833
FAX: (208) 334-3033

ILLINOIS
Region V
Illinois Department on Aging
421 E. Capitol Avenue
Suite 100
Springfield, Illinois 62701-1789
(217) 785-2870
Chicago office: (312) 814-2916
FAX: (217) 785-4477

INDIANA
Region V
Bureau of Aging and In-Home
    Services
Division of Disability, Aging and
    Rehabilitative Services
Family and Social Services
    Administration
402 W. Washington Street
Suite W454
P.O. Box 7083
Indianapolis, Indiana 46207-7083
(317) 232-7020
FAX: (317) 232-7867

IOWA
Region VII
Iowa Department of Elder Affairs
Clemens Building, Third Floor
200 Tenth Street
Des Moines, Iowa 50309-3609
(515) 281-4646
FAX: (515) 281-4036

KANSAS
Region VII
Department on Aging
New England Building
503 S. Kansas Avenue
Topeka, Kansas 66603-3404
(785) 296-4986
FAX: (785) 296-0256

KENTUCKY
Region IV
Office of Aging Services
Cabinet for Families and Children
Commonwealth of Kentucky
275 E. Main Street
Frankfort, Kentucky 40621
(502) 564-6930
FAX: (502) 564-4595

LOUISIANA
Region VI
Governor's Office of Elderly
  Affairs
P.O. Box 80374
Baton Rouge, Louisiana
  70898-0374
(504) 342-7100
FAX: (504) 342-7133

MAINE
Region I
Bureau of Elder and Adult
  Services
Department of Human Services
State House
Station 11
35 Anthony Avenue
Augusta, Maine 04333
(207) 624-5335
FAX: (207) 624-5361

MARYLAND
Region III
Maryland Office on Aging
State Office Building
Room 1007
301 W. Preston Street
Baltimore, Maryland 21201-2374
(410) 767-1100
FAX: (410) 333-7943
E-mail: sfw@mail.ooa.state.md.us

MASSACHUSETTS
Region I
Massachusetts Executive Office of
  Elder Affairs
One Ashburton Place, Fifth Floor
Boston, Massachusetts 02108
(617) 727-7750
FAX: (617) 727-9368

MICHIGAN
Region V
Michigan Office of Services to the
  Aging
N. Ottawa Tower, Third Floor
611 W. Ottawa
P.O. Box 30676
Lansing, Michigan 48909
(517) 373-8230
FAX: (517) 373-4092

MINNESOTA
Region V
Minnesota Board on Aging
444 Lafayette Road
St. Paul, Minnesota 55155-3843
(612) 297-7855
FAX: (612) 296-7855

MISSISSIPPI
Region IV
Division of Aging and Adult
    Services
750 N. State Street
Jackson, Mississippi 39202
(601) 359-4925
FAX: (601) 359-4370

MISSOURI
Region VII
Division on Aging
Department of Social Services
615 Howerton Court
P.O. Box 1337
Jefferson City, Missouri
    65102-1337
(573) 751-3082
FAX: (573) 751-8687

MONTANA
Region VIII
Senior and Long-Term Care
    Division
Department of Public Health and
    Human Services
111 Sanders
Room 211
P.O. Box 4210
Helena, Montana 59620
(406) 444-7788
FAX: (406) 444-7743

NEBRASKA
Region VII
Department of Health and
    Human Services
Division on Aging
1343 M Street
P.O. Box 95044
Lincoln, Nebraska 68509-5044
(402) 471-2307
FAX: (402) 471-4619

NEVADA
Region IX
Nevada Division for Aging
    Services
Department of Human Resources
State Mail Room Complex
340 N. Eleventh Street
Suite 203
Las Vegas, Nevada 89101
(702) 486-3545
FAX: (702) 486-3572

NEW HAMPSHIRE
Region I
Division of Elderly and Adult
    Services
State Office Park South
Brown Building, Suite 1
129 Pleasant Street
Concord, New Hampshire 03301
(603) 271-4680
FAX: (603) 271-4643

NEW JERSEY
Region II
Department of Health and Senior
  Services
New Jersey Division of Senior
  Affairs
P.O Box 807
Trenton, New Jersey 08625-0807
(609) 588-3141; 1-800-792-8820
FAX: (609) 588-3601

NEW MEXICO
Region VI
State Agency on Aging
La Villa Rivera Building
228 E. Palace Avenue,
  Ground Floor
Santa Fe, New Mexico 87501
(505) 827-7640
FAX: (505) 827-7649

NEW YORK
Region II
New York State Office for the
  Aging
2 Empire State Plaza
Albany, New York 12223-1251
(518) 474-5731; 1-800-342-9871
FAX: (518) 474-0608

NORTH CAROLINA
Region IV
Division of Aging
CB 29531
693 Palmer Drive
Raleigh, North Carolina
  27626-0531
(919) 733-3983
FAX: (919) 733-0443

NORTH DAKOTA
Region VIII
Department of Human Services
Aging Services Division
600 S. Second Street
Suite 1C
Bismarck, North Dakota 58504
(701) 328-8910
FAX: (701) 328-8989

NORTH MARIANA ISLANDS
Region IX
CNMI Office on Aging
P.O. Box 2178
Commonwealth of the Northern
  Mariana Islands
Saipan, Mariana Islands 96950
(670) 233-1320 or 1321
FAX: (670) 233-1327 or 0369

OHIO
Region V
Ohio Department of Aging
50 W. Broad Street
Ninth Floor
Columbus, Ohio 43215-5928
(614) 466-5500
FAX: (614) 466-5741

OKLAHOMA
Region VI
Aging Services Division
Department of Human Services
312 N.E. Twenty-Eighth Street
P.O. Box 25352
Oklahoma City, Oklahoma 73125
(405) 521-2281; (405) 521-2327
FAX: (405) 521-2086

OREGON
Region X
Senior and Disabled Services
  Division
500 Summer Street, N.E.,
  Second Floor
Salem, Oregon 97310-1015
(503) 945-5811
FAX: (503) 373-7823

PALAU
Region X
State Agency on Aging
Republic of Palau
Koror, Palau 96940
9-10-288-011-680-488-2736
FAX: 9-10-288-680-488-1662 or
  1597

PENNSYLVANIA
Region III
Pennsylvania Department of
  Aging
Commonwealth of Pennsylvania
555 Walnut Street, Fifth Floor
Harrisburg, Pennsylvania
  17101-1919
(717) 783-1550
FAX: (717) 772-3382

PUERTO RICO
Region II
Commonwealth of Puerto Rico
Governor's Office of Elderly
  Affairs
Call Box 50063
Old San Juan Station, Puerto Rico
  00902
(787) 721-5710;
  (787) 721-4560;
  (787) 721-6121
FAX: (787) 721-6510

RHODE ISLAND
Region I
Department of Elderly Affairs
160 Pine Street
Providence, Rhode Island
  02903-3708
(401) 277-2858
FAX: (401) 277-2130

AMERICAN SAMOA
Region IX
Territorial Administration on
  Aging
Government of American Samoa
Pago Pago, American Samoa
  96799
011-684-633-2207
FAX: 011-864-633-2533 or 633-
  7723

SOUTH CAROLINA
Region IV
Office of Senior and Long-Term
  Care Services
Department of Health and
  Human Services
P.O. Box 8206
Columbia, South Carolina
  29202-4535
(803) 898-2501
FAX: (803) 898-4515

SOUTH DAKOTA
Region VIII
Office of Adult Services and
  Aging
Richard F. Kneip Building
700 Governors Drive
Pierre, South Dakota 57501-2291
(605) 773-3656
FAX: (605) 773-6834

TENNESSEE
Region IV
Commission on Aging
Andrew Jackson Building,
    Ninth Floor
500 Deaderick Street
Nashville, Tennessee 37243-0860
(615) 741-2056
FAX: (615) 741-3309

TEXAS
Region VI
Texas Department on Aging
4900 N. Lamar, Fourth Floor
Austin, Texas 78751-2316
(512) 424-6840
FAX: (512) 424-6890

UTAH
Region VIII
Division of Aging and Adult
    Services
120 North 200 West
Box 45500
Salt Lake City, Utah 84145-0500
(801) 538-3910
FAX: (801) 538-4395

VERMONT
Region I
Vermont Department of Aging
    and Disabilities
Waterbury Complex
103 S. Main Street
Waterbury, Vermont 05671-2301
(802) 241-2400
FAX: (802) 241-2325

VIRGINIA
Region III
Virginia Department for the
    Aging
1600 Forest Avenue
Suite 102
Richmond, Virginia 23229
(804) 662-9333
FAX: (804) 662-9354

VIRGIN ISLANDS
Region II
Office of Senior Citizen Affairs
Virgin Islands Department of
    Human Services
Knud Hansen Complex,
    Building A
1303 Hospital Ground
Charlotte Amalie, Virgin Islands
    00802
(340) 774-0930
FAX: (340) 774-3466

WASHINGTON
Region X
Aging and Adult Services
    Administration
Department of Social & Health
    Services
P.O. Box 45050
Olympia, Washington
    98504-5050
(360) 493-2500
FAX: (360) 438-8633

WEST VIRGINIA
Region III
West Virginia Bureau of Senior
    Services
Holly Grove, Building 10
1900 Kanawha Boulevard East
Charleston, West Virginia 25305
(304) 558-3317
FAX: (304) 558-0004

WISCONSIN
Region V
Bureau of Aging and Long-Term
    Care Resources
Department of Health and Family
    Services
P.O. Box 7851
Madison, Wisconsin 53707
(608) 266-2536
FAX: (608) 267-3203

WYOMING
Region VIII
Office on Aging
Department of Health
117 Hathaway Building
Room 139
Cheyenne, Wyoming 82002-0710
(307) 777-7986
FAX: (307) 777-5340

State Hospice Organizations

ALABAMA
Alabama Hospice Organization
(334) 213-7944

ALASKA
Hospice of Anchorage
(907) 561-5322

ARIZONA
Arizona Hospice Organization
(602) 704-0210

ARKANSAS
Arkansas State Hospice
  Association
(870) 862-0337

CALIFORNIA
California State Hospice
  Association
(916) 441-3770

COLORADO
Colorado Hospice Organization
(303) 449-1142

CONNECTICUT
Hospice Council of Connecticut
(860) 233-2222

DELAWARE
Delaware Hospice, Inc.
1-800-838-9800

FLORIDA
Florida Hospices and Palliative
  Care, Inc.
(850) 878-2632

GEORGIA
Georgia Hospice Organization
(770) 924-6073

HAWAII
Hawaii State Hospice Network
(808) 924-9255

IDAHO
Idaho Hospice Organization
(208) 726-8464

ILLINOIS
Illinois State Hospice
   Organization
(773) 324-8844

INDIANA
Indiana Hospice Organization
(317) 338-4041

IOWA
Iowa Hospice Organization
(515) 243-1046

KANSAS
Association of Kansas Hospices
(316) 263-6380

KENTUCKY
Kentucky Association of Hospices
(888) 322-7317

LOUISIANA
Louisiana Hospice Organization
(504) 945-2414

MARYLAND
Hospice Network of Maryland
(410) 729-4571

MASSACHUSETTS
Hospice Federation of
   Massachusetts
(781) 255-7077

MICHIGAN
Michigan Hospice Organization
(517) 886-6667

MINNESOTA
Minnesota Hospice Organization
(651) 659-0423

MISSISSIPPI
Mississippi Hospice Organization
(601) 236-1459

MISSOURI
Missouri Hospice Organization
(816) 350-7702

MONTANA
Montana Hospice Organization
(406) 248-7442

NEBRASKA
Nebraska Hospice Association
(308) 687-6065

NEVADA
Hospice Association of Nevada
(702) 796-3134

NEW HAMPSHIRE
New Hampshire Hospice
   Organization
(603) 228-9870

NEW JERSEY
New Jersey Hospice and Palliative
   Care Organization
(908) 233-0060

NEW MEXICO
Texas and New Mexico Hospice
   Organization
(512) 454-1247

NEW YORK
New York State Hospice
  Association
(518) 446-1483

NORTH CAROLINA
Hospice for the Carolinas
(919) 878-1717

NORTH DAKOTA
North Dakota Hospice
  Organization
(701) 774-7400

OHIO
Ohio Hospice Organization
(614) 274-9513

OKLAHOMA
Hospice Association of Oklahoma
(918) 835-6742

OREGON
Oregon Hospice Association
(503) 228-2104

PENNSYLVANIA
Pennsylvania Hospice Network
(717) 230-9993

RHODE ISLAND
Rhode Island State Hospice
  Organization
(401) 788-0811

SOUTH CAROLINA
Hospice for the Carolinas
(803) 791-4220

SOUTH DAKOTA
South Dakota Hospice
  Organization
(605) 664-9371

TENNESSEE
Tennessee Hospice Organization
1-800-638-6411

TEXAS
Texas and New Mexico Hospice
  Organization
(512) 454-1247

UTAH
Utah Hospice Organization
(801) 321-5661

VERMONT
Hospice Council of Vermont
(802) 229-0579

VIRGINIA
Virginia Association for Hospices
(540) 686-6448

WASHINGTON
Washington State Hospice
  Organization
(509) 456-0438

WEST VIRGINIA
Hospice Council of West Virginia
(304) 529-4217

WISCONSIN
Hospice Organization of
  Wisconsin
(608) 233-7166

WYOMING
Wyoming Hospice Organization
(307) 632-3761

PUERTO RICO
Puerto Rico Home Health and
  Hospice Association
(787) 758-8180

Long-Term Care Ombudsman and State Survey Agencies

The Long-Term Care Ombudsman investigates complaints against nursing homes, acts as an advocate for residents, and mediates disputes between nursing homes and residents or their families. The Ombudsman is the only independent person in the regulatory system; the sole concern of these offices is to protect the rights and well-being of residents. They stand ready to help if you need information on the nursing homes in your state, or if you have a complaint about one of those nursing homes.

If you are considering placement, you should call the Office of the Long-Term Care Ombudsman in your state for information on the quality of care in the facility you are considering.

State survey agencies conduct an annual survey and inspection of every Medicare- or Medicaid-certified nursing home in their state. They cite homes for deficient practices. Because these agencies enforce federal guidelines on nursing homes, they have the power to sanction homes.

If you have a complaint about the quality of life or quality of care inside a nursing home, contact your state's survey agency as well as your Ombudsman.

	Ombudsman	*Survey Agency*
Alabama	(334) 242-5743	(334) 240-3503
Alaska	(907) 563-6393	(907) 561-8081
Arizona	(602) 542-4446	(602) 255-1177
Arkansas	(501) 682-2441	(501) 682-8430
California	(916) 323-6681	(916) 445-3054
Colorado	(303) 722-0300	(303) 692-2835
Connecticut	(203) 424-5200	(203) 566-1073
Delaware	(302) 453-3820	(302) 577-6666
District of Columbia	(202) 662-4933	(202) 727-7190
Florida	(904) 488-6190	(904) 487-2527
Georgia	(404) 657-5319	(404) 657-5850
Hawaii	(808) 586-0100	(808) 586-4080
Idaho	(208) 334-2220	(208) 334-6626
Illinois	(217) 785-3143	(217) 782-2913
Indiana	(317) 232-7134	(317) 383-6262
Iowa	(515) 281-5187	(515) 281-4115
Kansas	(913) 296-6539	(913) 296-1240
Kentucky	(502) 564-6930	(502) 562-2800

(continued)

Long-Term Care Ombudsman and State Survey Agencies

	Ombudsman	*Survey Agency*
Louisiana	(504) 925-1700	(504) 240-3517
Maine	(207) 621-1079	(207) 287-2606
Maryland	(410) 225-1074	(410) 764-2750
Massachusetts	(617) 727-7750	(617) 727-5860
Michigan	(517) 336-6753	(517) 335-8649
Minnesota	(612) 296-0382	(612) 643-2171
Mississippi	(601) 359-4970	(601) 354-7300
Missouri	(573) 751-3082	(573) 751-6302
Montana	(406) 444-5900	(406) 444-2037
Nebraska	(402) 471-2306	(402) 471-4961
Nevada	(702) 486-3545	(702) 687-4475
New Hampshire	(603) 271-4375	(603) 271-4592
New Jersey	(609) 984-7831	(609) 292-9874
New Mexico	(505) 827-7663	(505) 827-4200
New York	(518) 474-0108	(518) 473-3517
North Carolina	(919) 733-3983	(919) 733-7461
North Dakota	(701) 224-2577	(701) 224-2352
Ohio	(614) 644-7922	(614) 466-7857
Oklahoma	(405) 521-6734	(405) 271-4200
Oregon	(503) 378-6533	(503) 945-6456
Pennsylvania	(717) 783-7247	(717) 787-8015

(continued)

	Ombudsman	*Survey Agency*
Rhode Island	(401) 277-2858	(401) 277-2566
South Carolina	(803) 737-7500	(803) 737-7205
South Dakota	(605) 773-3656	(605) 773-3356
Tennessee	(615) 741-2056	(615) 367-6316
Texas	(512) 438-2633	(512) 834-3053
Utah	(801) 538-3924	(801) 538-6559
Vermont	(802) 748-8721	(802) 277-2345
Virginia	(804) 644-2923	(804) 367-2100
Washington	(206) 838-6810	(206) 493-2560
West Virginia	(304) 558-3317	(304) 558-0050
Wisconsin	(608) 266-8944	(608) 267-7185
Wyoming	(307) 322-5553	(307) 777-7123
Puerto Rico	(809) 721-8225	(809) 721-4050
American Samoa	(684) 633-1222	
Guam	(671) 734-7210	

Alternative Resources to Enhance Home Life

Aromatherapy

There is probably nothing as soothing in a sick room as the use of essential oils. Pure lavender oil is said to bring peace. Both lemon and orange oils are said to raise the spirits. Geranium oil is said to inspire courage and hope in difficult situations.

I believe that a wealth of comfort may be obtained from these unspoiled elements of nature's bounty. These inexpensive luxuries are easy to use and have no side effects. Usually even people who are chemically sensitive respond well to essential oils.

One of the best and most trustworthy suppliers I have come across is

Liberty Naturals
8120 S.E. Stark Street
Portland, Oregon 97215
1-800-289-8427

Call for their catalog. Their prices are low, and they have the equipment, such as diffusers and lamps, you need. They sell wholesale, as long as you meet their minimum order requirement, about fifty dollars.

The best book on using aromatherapy is undoubtedly Valerie Worwood's *Complete Book of Essential Oils and Aromatherapy,* published by New World Library. Dr. Worwood's book is thorough, easy to read, and full of suggestions for the use of essential oils to alleviate all sorts of conditions—from bedsores to headaches to anxiety.

Essential oils are starting to be used even in mainstream medicine. Leicester Hospital, in Leicester, England, uses diffused oil of lavender at night instead of giving its patients sleeping pills.

Instructional Audio and Video Tapes

A wonderful resource for topical audio and video tapes helpful to both caregivers and their patients is

Sounds True
1-800-333-9185

They have over two hundred titles recorded by some of today's most compelling scholars and teachers. Many explore spiritual practices from a number of traditions—Jewish, Christian, Buddhist, Hindu, and Sufi, for example.

The following are some of my favorites:

Audio

Meditation
Awakening Compassion, by Pema Chodron
The Art of Forgiving, by Robin Casarjian
The Art of Mindful Living, by Thich Nhat Hanh
Meditation for Beginners, by Jack Kornfeld

Aging
Conscious Aging, by Ram Dass
How to Never Grow Old and Die Young at Heart, by Bernie Siegal
The Good Life of Helen Nearing, by Helen Nearing

Dying
Final Wisdom: What the Dying Can Teach Us About Living
A Year to Live, by Stephen Levine
Tibetan Wisdom for Living and Dying, by Sogyal Rinpoche
Rituals for Conscious Dying, by David Feinstein

Health and Healing
Break Through Pain, by Shinzen Young
Healing with Great Music, by Don Campbell
Healthy Breathing, by Ken Cohen

Caring for Yourself
When Things Fall Apart, by Pema Chodron
Humor and Healing, by Bernie Siegal
Homeopathic Healing, by Dana Ullman

Video

Gentle Exercise
Meditative Movements, by Thich Nhat Hanh
Qigong, by Ken Cohen

Meditation
The Inner Art of Meditation, by Jack Kornfeld
Secular Meditation, by the Dalai Lama

Aging
How to Never Grow Old and Die Young at Heart, by Bernie Siegal

Glossary of Terms

ACETYLCHOLINE: a chemical that acts as a neurotransmitter; an imbalance between dopamine and acetylcholine may lead to Parkinsonian symptoms.

AGONIST: a drug that increases neurotransmitter activity by stimulating the dopamine receptors directly.

AKINESIA: little or no movement.

ANTICHOLINERGIC DRUG: a drug that blocks the action of acetylcholine; used to restore the balance between acetylcholine and dopamine.

BRADYKINESIA: slowness of movement.

COGWHEEL RIGIDITY: muscular rigidity that produces a ratcheted resistance in the limbs of Parkinson's patients or persons taking certain antipsychotic medications.

DEMENTIA: a mental disorder involving loss of intellectual abilities, including impairment of memory and judgment.

DOPAMINE: a neurotransmitter that regulates movement, balance, and walking; 80 percent of dopamine is lost before symptoms of Parkinson's disease appear.

DYSKINESIA: involuntary movement, usually as a side effect of medication.

DYSTONIA: ongoing contraction or spasm in a group of muscles.

FESTINATION: a tendency to take short, accelerating steps in walking.

FREEZING: a temporary inability to move, often when in doorways or narrow spaces but sometimes of unknown cause.

LEVODOPA: a chemical that is converted to dopamine by the enzyme dopa decarboxylase.

MICROGRAPHIA: small, cramped handwriting.

NEUROTRANSMITTER: a chemical substance that carries impulses from one nerve cell to another.

ON–OFF EFFECTS: changes in a patient's ability to move or perform while on medications; sometimes occur abruptly, and often at unpredictable times.

ORTHOSTATIC HYPOTENSION: a decrease in blood pressure upon standing; may be related to certain drugs.

PARKINSONISM: a clinical condition that usually involves tremor, rigidity, and bradykinesia.

PLAQUES AND TANGLES: term applied to the abnormal brain cells seen upon autopsy, often but not always associated with Alzheimer's disease.

RIGIDITY: stiffness in the limbs and muscles.

SUNDOWNING: agitation observed in some Alzheimer's patients in the late afternoon.

TREMOR: involuntary shaking; in Parkinson's, usually of a limb at rest.

Bibliography

Aging

Berman, H. *Interpreting the Aging Self.* New York: Springer, 1994.

Bianchi, E. *Aging as a Spiritual Journey.* New York: Crossroad, 1989.

Caregiving

Benson, H. *The Relaxation Response.* New York: Morrow, 1975.

Dunn, H. *Hard Choices for Loving People: CPR, Artificial Feeding, Comfort Measures Only and the Elderly Patient.* Herndon, VA: A & A, 1994.

Gray-Davidson, F. *The Alzheimer's Sourcebook.* Chicago: Contemporary Books/McGraw-Hill. (A guide to looking after a person with Alzheimer's; focuses especially on communication issues.)

——— *Alzheimer's Disease FAQ: Making Sense of the Journey.* Chicago: Contemporary Books/McGraw-Hill, 1998. (An alternative take on, and practical guide to, Alzheimer's; focuses especially on the issue of dementia.)

Kirsta, A. *The Book of Stress Survival.* New York: Simon & Schuster, 1987.

Lidell, L. *The Book of Massage.* New York: Simon & Schuster, 1984.

Ray, M.C. *I'm Here to Help: A Guide for Caregivers.* New York: Bantam, 1997. (Excellent attitude training; easy to read, with insightful suggestions related to the care of the seriously ill.)

Reoch, R. *To Die Well.* San Francisco: Harper Collins, 1996. (Perhaps the best general book on self-help in caregiving, utilizing alternative do-it-yourself therapies in a simple, thorough way.)

Worwood, Valerie. *Complete Book of Essential Oils and Aromatherapy.* Novato, CA: New World Library, 1981.

Death and Dying

Duda, D. *Coming Home: A Guide to Dying at Home.* New York: Aurora Press, 1987. (Excellent, sensible, how-to guide to caring for an ill person. Useful whether the illness is terminal or not. Includes spiritual lessons.)

Kübler-Ross, E., M.D. *On Death and Dying.* New York: Macmillan, 1969.

———— *Questions and Answers on Death and Dying.* New York: Macmillan, 1974.

Levine, S. *Who Dies?* New York: Doubleday, 1982.

Longaker, C. *Facing Death and Finding Hope.* New York: Doubleday, 1997.

Moody, R., M.D. *Life After Life.* New York: Bantam, 1988.

Reimer, J. *Jewish Reflections on Death.* New York: Schocken, 1974.

Grief

Forman, P.K. *After You Say Good-Bye: When Someone You Love Dies of AIDS.* San Francisco: Chronicle Books, 1992.

Kraus, P. *Why Me? Coping with Grief, Loss, and Change.* New York: Bantam, 1988.

Rando, T. *How to Go on Living When Someone You Love Dies.* San Francisco: Chronicle Books, 1992.

Volkan, V. *Life After Loss: The Lessons of Grief.* New York: Collier, 1994.

Illness

Acherberg, J. *Imagery in Healing.* Boston: Shambhala, 1985.

Cousins, N. *Anatomy of an Illness.* New York: Norton, 1979.

———— *The Healing Heart.* New York: Norton, 1983.

Illich, I. *Medical Nemesis.* New York: Pantheon, 1976.

Medical Practice and Aging

Callahan, D. *Setting Limits: Medical Goals in an Aging Society.* New York: Simon & Schuster, 1987.

Murphy, D., M.D. *Honest Medicine: Shattering the Myths About Aging and Health Care.* The Atlantic Monthly Press, 1994.

Planning Ahead

Budish, A. *Avoiding the Medicaid Trap: How Every American Can Beat the Catastrophic Costs of Nursing Home Care.* New York: Avon, 1981.

Spiritual

Dalai Lama. *Kindness, Clarity, and Insight.* New York: Snow Lion, 1984.

Dass, R. *How Can I Help?* New York: Knopf, 1985.

Dossey, L., M.D. *Recovering the Soul.* New York: Bantam, 1989.

Frankl, V. *Man's Search for Meaning.* New York: Simon & Schuster, 1959.

Hanh, T. N.. *Being Peace.* Berkeley, CA: Parallax Press, 1987.

Jampolsy, G., M.D. *Good-Bye to Guilt.* New York: Bantam, 1985.

Kushner, H. *When Bad Things Happen to Good People.* New York: Schocken, 1981.

Rinpoche, S. *Tibetan Book of Living and Dying.* San Francisco: Harper Collins, 1997.

Index

advance medical directives
  explained, 89
  extending life, wishes
    regarding, 89–90
aging, state agencies on, 131–39
AIDS and HIV
  adrenal insufficiency and low
    hormone production, 37
  infections associated with, 37
  precautions for caregivers, 36
  transmitting disease, 36
AIDS and HIV, fighting fatigue
  body's compensation for, 40
  forms of fatigue, 39–40
AIDS and HIV, lifestyle and
    fatigue
  anxiety and depression, 41
  exercise and weight lifting, 40
  sleeping problems, dealing
    with, 40–41
AIDS and HIV, medical
    management
  anemia, HIV drugs causing,
    37–38
  anti-inflammatory drugs, 38
AIDS and HIV, nutrition
  loss of appetite, reasons for, 38

nausea, vomiting, and diarrhea,
    strategies for, 39
  nutritional deficiencies and
    dietary changes, 38
  strategies for loss of appetite, 39
Alzheimer's disease
  caring for caregiver, support
    groups, 46–47
  described, 43–44
  diagnosing, 44
Alzheimer's disease, the challenge
    for caregivers
  caregiver's duties, 44
  communicating with
    patient, 45
  family caregivers and stress in
    patient, 46
  protecting and helping patient
    stay occupied, 45
  recognizing fears and losing
    sense of taste, 46
American Association of Retired
    Persons (AARP), consulting
    and long-term care
    insurance, 82–83
Area Agencies on Aging (AAAs),
    131–39

aromatherapy
  essential oils and suppliers, 150
  Liberty Naturals, 150
assets, transfer of
  asset exemption, 77–78
  Medicaid eligibility, 77
  transfers between spouses or
    unmarried couples, 78
audio and video tapes,
    instructional
  audio, 151
  Sounds True, 150
  video, 151

cancer, physical problems
  morphine, 42
  nausea and pain, 41–42
  nutrition, maintaining proper, 42
  treatments, side effects from, 41
cancer, psychological problems
  cancer support group and
    becoming a confidant, 43
  depression and passivity, 43
  fear of untimely death, 42
  optimism, anger, and denial,
    42–43
caregiver, caring for
  checklist for, 26–27
  depression, example of, 18–19
  emotional issues, dealing with,
    18
  exercise, 21–22
  fatigue, knowing warning signs,
    23
  feeling overwhelmed, 19
  flexibility, 19
  forgetting about yourself, 18
  nutrition, 21
  proper breathing, 22–23
  safety precautions, 22

sleep, 20–21
  unconscious abusers, 17
  unresolved issues, 17
caregiver, emotional health of
  anger, dealing with, 24
  emotional reactions to
    situations, 23–24
  sense of humor, retaining, 24
caregiver, handling grief
  caring for yourself, suggestions
    for, 25–26
  giving way to grief, 24
  Internet support, 25
  sharing your pain and spiritual
    practice, 25
  taking a break, suggestions
    before leaving, 26
caregiver, hiring professional
  agency, questions for, 61
  individual caregiver, questions
    for, 62
caregiver, knowing what to do
  being overwhelmed and getting
    help, 19–20
  special equipment, 20
caregiver education
  caregiver organizations,
    124–25
  death and dying, 125–26
  illnesses, diseases, disabilities,
    122–24
caregiver's responsibilities
  burnout, 100
  wages and compensation, 99
  work expected and hours,
    defining, 99–100
caregiving
  accepting challenge of, 4–7
  becoming tainted, 3
  caregiving education, need for, 4

caring about yourself, 2
caring for caregiver, 17–27
comfort levels, establishing,
    12–13
daily problem solving, 7–10
developing plan, 10–11
emotional comfort, 13–14
forgotten skills, reasons for,
    2–3
making home safe, 15–16
patient checklist, 16–17
society's need for, 2
where to begin, 1
caregiving, accepting challenge of
caregiving and martyrdom, 4–5
death, 6
getting knowledge for coping, 5
heroism, 7
hidden rewards, 6
Public Guardian, 5
self-destructive sacrifice, 4
*Complete Book of Essential Oils
    and Aromatherapy*
    (Worwood), 150

death
caregiver's role and slow
    periods, 102–3
checklist when patient is dying,
    108–9
death away from home, 104–5
deciding where to die, 101
dying process, 105–8
grieving, 109–10
hospice home nurses, 102
predeath vigil, 103
romanticizing and denial, 102
death away from home
dying in hospice or nursing
    home, 104

hospice in nursing homes, 105
making patient comfortable, 105
nursing homes, policy for dying
    patients, 104
doctor
choice of physician, questions
    when deciding, 53–54
equipment, services, and using
    nurses and staff, 54–55
knowing needs at doctor's
    visit, 54
patient's insurance, Medicaid,
    or Medicare, 54
dying process
afterlife and patient's
    appearance, 107
caregiver as peaceful human
    presence, 105
leaving family and deeply
    conscious patients, 107–8
losing heat and death rattle,
    106–7
old family business, taking care
    of, 105
power of choice and eating and
    drinking less, 105–6
when patient stops eating and
    reducing medication, 106

elder abuse
abuse in nursing home, what to
    do, 98
imminent danger, what to
    do, 98
signs of possible abuse, 97–98
emotional comfort
being hopeful and never
    assuming worst, 14
feeling overwhelmed, finding
    solutions for, 14

emotional comfort *(continued)*
  level of, 13
  patient's condition, affects on
    behavior, 14
  spiritual issues, approaching,
    13–14
entitlement programs
  COBRA, Hill-Burton program,
    and Pharmaceutical Indigent
    programs, 71
  eligibility guidelines, 70
  food stamps, Home Energy
    Assistance Program (HEAP),
    Weatherization Referral and
    Packaging Program
    (WRAP), 72
  Social Security and
    Supplemental Security
    Income (SSI), 70–71
  Veterans Benefits and replacing
    lost income, 71
essential oils. *See* aromatherapy

grieving
  blaming yourself, 109–10
  tidal wave of grief and rash
    decisions, 109

health care, paying for
  entitlement programs, 70–72
  excess income program, 78
  HMO or managed health care
    plan, choosing, 80–81
  home- and community-based
    waivers, 76–77
  Medicaid, 75–76
  Medicare, 72–73
  Medicare HMO, 73–74
  Medigap, 73

money, other sources of, 84–86
  private assets, other ways of
    protecting, 79–80
  private insurance, 82–84
  spousal impoverishment, 78–79
  supplemental coverage, 74
  system, navigating, 77
  transfer of assets, 77–78
heart disease
  angina, explained, 50
  heart attack symptoms, 51
  heart failure, signs and
    symptoms of, 50–51
HMO or managed care plan,
    choosing
  access to specialists and
    preventive care, 80
  choice of doctors and other
    providers, 80
  extent of service area and other
    benefits, 81
  total cost and review
    process, 81
HMOs and hospitals
  advantages of, 55
  HMOs, shortcomings of, 55
  hospital health professionals, 56
home- and community-based
    waivers
  advantages of, 76
  flexibility of state for designing
    program, 76–77
  services utilized under waiver
    program, 76
home health services
  caregivers, hiring from agencies
    and directly, 58. *See also*
    caregiver, hiring professional
  explained, 57

fees and finding help, 58
nutritionists, therapists, and
home health aides, 57–58
private care managers, 58–59
registered nurses (RNs), physicians, and social workers, 57
home safety checklist
floors and stairs, 15
kitchen and bathroom, 15–16
outside and security systems, 16
hospice (palliative care)
explained, 59
getting the best, 59–60
organizations, state, 141–43

in-home services. *See* services,
finding in-home
intensive home care. *See* long-term
care, common conditions
Internet resources, 127–30

Kübler-Ross, Elizabeth *(On Death
and Dying)*, 8

legal documents
advance medical directories,
89–90
medical power of attorney, 90
trusts and setting up plan,
91–92
wills and financial power of
attorney, 90
Liberty Naturals, 150
long-term care, common
conditions requiring
AIDS and HIV, 36–41
Alzheimer's disease, 43–47
cancer, 41–43
heart disease, 50–51

Parkinson's disease, 29–36
stroke, 47–50
long-term care and patient's
rights, 93–97
long-term care ombudsman
explained, 145–46
nursing home complaints,
146–48

Medicaid
benefits and personal care
services, 75–76
explained, 75
Medicare
coverage, 72–73
explained, 72
Medicare HMO, 73–74
Medigap, 73
mental health services, questions
when deciding
government benefits, qualifying
for, 61
insurance coverage, 60–61
location of service, 60
money for care, other sources of
funds and foundations, 86
IRAs, 86
life insurance policies, 85
reverse mortgages, 84–85

nursing home, choosing
activities program, religious
observances, and social
services, 66
cleanliness and day room, 64
dining room, food services, and
kitchen, 64
financial considerations and
residents' rights, 67–68

nursing home *(continued)*
  fire safety and bedrooms, 63
  grooming and laundry, 66
  isolation room and grounds, 65
  licensing and certification, 62
  location and accident
    prevention, 62–63
  medical services and nursing
    services, 65
  special considerations and
    staff, 67
  toilet and bathing facilities,
    63–64

Omnibus Budget Reconciliation
  Act (OBRA), 93–96
On Death and Dying (Kübler-
  Ross), 8

palliative care. *See* hospice
Parkinsonism
  described, 30–31
  medications for, 31
Parkinson's disease
  checklist for patient, 34–36
  classic signs of, 30
  counseling and support
    groups, 32
  described, 29–30
  falls and injuries, 32
  intermittent tremors and motor
    deficits, 31
Parkinsonism, 30–31
  symptom variations, 31
Parkinson's disease, medical
  management
  Amantadine (Symmetrel), 32
  drug prolonging action of
    Levodopa, 33
  dyskinesia, 33

Levodopa (L-dopa), 32
  tremor medications and side
    effects, 33
Parkinson's disease, nutritional
  guidelines
  digestive system, 33
  protein intake and maintaining
    weight, 34
  Sinemet, 33–34
  supplements and dehydra-
    tion, 34
patient's legal rights
  items and services not charged
    to resident, 96
  nursing facility, rights of
    residents, 94–96
  nursing home charges to
    residents, 96–97
  Omnibus Budget Reconcil-
    iation Act (OBRA) and
    long-term care facilities,
    required services, 93–96
  respecting, 92–93
  violating rights in long-term
    care, 93
plan, developing
  death care, discussing with
    doctor, 10–11
  description of medical
    difficulty, 11
  new medical problems and
    physical equipment, getting
    help with, 11
  patient file, what to include, 10
plan, setting up
  extra copies, 92
  legal documents, distributing
    copies of, 91
predeath vigil
  help from second person, 103

planning for needs and final
stages, 103
private insurance
American Association of
Retired Persons (AARP),
consulting and long-term
care insurance, 82–83
checking rating publications, 84
family health profile, study-
ing, 83
getting most from policy, 82
policies, examining a few,
83–84
problem solving, daily
accepting your emotions,
seeking therapy, 9
adaptability, 7
being well informed about
disease, examples, 9–10
emotional stages of seriously ill,
understanding, 8
having plan, 7
illness, examples of accepting,
8–9
professional resources
the doctor, 53–55
HMOs and hospitals, 55–56
home health services, 57–59
hospice, 59–60
mental health services, 60–61
nursing home, choosing, 62–68
pharmacists, 56–57
professional caregiver, hiring,
61–62

resources, alternative
aromatherapy, 149–150
instructional audio and video
tapes, 150-51
responsibility, legal

advance planning and legally
defining responsibility,
87–88
caregiver's responsibilities,
99–100
court-appointed guardian and
finances of incapacitated
parent, 88
elder abuse, 97–98
legal documents, 89–92
legal plans for future, 88
patient's legal rights, 92–97
reluctance of elderly person, 89
reverse mortgages
debt, paying off, 85
explained, 84
HECM (Home Equity
Conversion Mortgage),
qualifying for federally
insured, 85
how to get, 84

services, finding in-home
health and education, 118–19
hospice, 119
in-home services and general
information, 112–18
state survey agencies
explained, 145–46
nursing home complaints,
146–48
stroke
bathroom habits and sex
drive, 48
chewing, swallowing, and
blood clots, 49
fear, anxiety, and depression,
49–50
high blood pressure and time
to heal, 49

stroke *(continued)*
  normal movement, recover-
    ing, 48
  positive thinking, 50
  speech, 47–48
  vision problems, 47
  what happens afterwards, 47

supplemental coverage
  explained, 74
  joining a plan, considerations
    before, 74

Worwood, Valerie *(Complete Book
    of Essential Oils and
    Aromatherapy)*, 150